4 MONTHS to a 4 HOUR MARATHON

4 MONTHS to a 4 HOUR MARATHON

David Kuehls

A Perigee Book

THE BERKLEY PUBLISHING GROUP
Published by the Penguin Group
Penguin Group (USA) Inc.
375 Hudson Street, New York, New York 10014, USA
Penguin Group (Canada), 90 Eglinton Avenue East, Suite 700, Toronto, Ontario M4P 2Y3, Canada
(a division of Pearson Penguin Canada Inc.)
Penguin Books Ltd., 80 Strand, London WC2R 0RL, England
Penguin Group Ireland, 25 St. Stephen's Green, Dublin 2, Ireland (a division of Penguin Books Ltd.)
Penguin Group (Australia), 250 Camberwell Road, Camberwell, Victoria 3124, Australia
(a division of Pearson Australia Group Pty. Ltd.)
Penguin Books India Pvt. Ltd., 11 Community Centre, Panchsheel Park, New Delhi—110 017, India
Penguin Group (NZ), Cnr. Airborne and Rosedale Roads, Albany, Auckland 1310, New Zealand
(a division of Pearson New Zealand Ltd.)
Penguin Books (South Africa) (Pty.) Ltd., 24 Sturdee Avenue, Rosebank, Johannesburg 2196,
South Africa

Penguin Books Ltd., Registered Offices: 80 Strand, London WC2R 0RL, England

PRINTING HISTORY
First Perigee trade paperback edition / July 1998
Updated Perigee trade paperback edition / July 2006

Updated Perigee trade paperback ISBN: 0-399-53259-5

The Library of Congress has cataloged the first Perigee edition as follows:

Kuehls, Dave.
    Four months to a four-hour marathon / Dave Kuehls. — 1st ed.
        p.   cm.
    "A Perigee Book."
    ISBN 0-399-52415-0
    1. Marathon running—Training.   I. Title
GV1065.17.T73K84   1998
796.42'52—dc21
                                                            97-40763
                                                            CIP

PRINTED IN THE UNITED STATES OF AMERICA

10   9   8   7   6

Outdoor recreational activities are by their very nature potentially hazardous. All participants in such
activities must assume the responsibility for their own actions and safety. If you have any health
problems or medical conditions, consult with your physician before undertaking any outdoor activities.
The information contained in this guidebook cannot replace sound judgment and good decision-
making, which can help reduce risk exposure, nor does the scope of this book allow for disclosure of all
the potential hazards and risks involved in such activities.

Learn as much as possible about the outdoor recreational activities in which you participate, prepare for
the unexpected, and be cautious. The reward will be a safer and more enjoyable experience.

CONTENTS

INTRODUCTION: WHY 4 HOURS? AND WHY 4 MONTHS?

The genesis for this book came from two events. The first occured in the late 1980s when my father, Ernie Kuehls, picked up running. He was a 50-something math professor who hadn't run at all in his life. In fact, he hadn't participated in sports for more than 25 years. He was a bit overweight and—he soon found out—he had no endurance at all.

Yet one day he headed out the door for a run.

My dad didn't make half a mile.

But he kept at it. After a while he ran a mile without stopping. Then 2 miles, then 4 miles.

One event loomed in the back of his mind.

That event was the marathon.

As a goal for his first marathon Ernie chose a specific time goal. The goal was **to break 4 hours**. And he chose a specific time frame in which to train for that marathon: **4 months**, the optimal time to train for a marathon—because any longer and you're likely to be burned out on training. Any less and you're not prepared.

And after **4 months** of training my dad completed his first marathon in under **4 hours** (3 hours and 58 minutes, to be exact).

Flash forward a few years. I'm standing at the finish chute of the 1993 New York City Marathon on assignment for *Runner's World* magazine. I'm writing an article about the blanket crew who supply some 25,000 finishers with shiny, heat-retaining blankets. As I stand at the finish chute and watch the runners come in, first a trickle at just over 2 hours, then more toward 3 hours and, finally, at **4 hours** they're crossing like a St. Patrick's Day parade, I come to a realization: **most** of the marathon runners out there are **just like my dad.** They're out there to run a marathon and **4 hours is the goal.**

THE 4 STEPS TO A 4-HOUR MARATHON

1. Train smartly.

2. Eat effectively.

3. Rest wisely.

4. Pick a fast marathon.

Why? Because **4 hours is a doable goal.** You don't need tons of speed (which is the hardest part of running to come by), just a goodly amount of endurance (something everyone can build into their system, just like my dad). In addition, there is something quasi-mystical about the **4-hour marathon.** A "foot populi" version of what surrounded the 4-minute mile for half a dozen fleet-footed milers back in the 1950s.

So I decided to write a book. This book.

I decided I would tell **4-hour marathoners** exactly what to wear, what to eat, how to train and how to run the marathon.

Every sentence would be geared toward one goal: Getting the reader to the finish line of a **marathon** in **4 hours.**

And to help me with the book, what better person than my dad, who set out to do—and did—just what you're about to learn—and do—from reading this book.

In **4 months,** you too can run a **4-hour marathon.**

Read on.

OTHER THINGS THAT TAKE 4 HOURS

A round of golf
Extra-innings baseball game
Preparing Thanksgiving dinner
Afternoon classes
Dinner and a movie

one

BASIC TRAINING

Running Form

Running is the easiest exercise to master. You don't need much balance, like you do for riding a bicycle. And you don't need a couple hundred bucks and good arm-leg coordination, like you do for cross-country skiing. Or coordination, for aerobics. Or patience, for walking. Or gills, for swimming.

You just need to get out the door and do what you did when you were a kid—run.

But many young adults and older adults have forgotten what it was like to run the way they did when they were seven or eight. They look like they've been stuck behind an office desk or school desk or plopped on a couch for too long. And they probably have been.

So here are a few pointers on running form—as you begin training for a **4-hour marathon**—for the kid in all of us.

Let's start from the top:

1 Your head: Should be straight up and down or slightly leaning forward. If your head is arching back, you throw the rest of your body backward.

2 Your mouth: Breathe through a comfortably open mouth. Some runners like to breathe in through the nose, then out through the mouth. But unless you're running through a cloud of black flies, why not open your mouth and suck in all the oxygen you can get?

3 The lower lip: Loose. If you have a loose lower lip that means you're not clenching your teeth. And the rest of your body is staying loose too.

4 Shoulders: Low rather than high. Loose rather than tense. They should have an upright or slight forward lean.

5 Arms: Bent perpendicular at the elbow. Swing back and forth between the waist and the bottom of your rib cage— try to do as little side-to-side motion as possible. Give yourself a couple inches berth on each side so you're not punching yourself in the kidneys with each swing.

6 Hands: Half-fists. Do not clench. Keep them between waist level and rib-cage level for most of your running. Your arm cadence should mimic your stride. Pump them higher and harder when sprinting or going up hills.

7 Thumbs: Keep loose and outside the fist.

8 Back: Upright or slight forward lean.

9 Chest: Upright.

10 Lungs: Learn to belly breathe, that is, take deep breaths and push down with your diaphragm, expanding the

stomach, not the chest. This ensures that you are inflating the lungs with each breath.

11 Hips: Forward and under you.

12 Butt: Forward and tucked under.

13 Knees: Gentle lift but not pronounced. You should not feel your knees lift in the thigh muscles, unless you are running uphill or sprinting.

14 Leg swing: Reach out just ahead of you to land, and swing your leg back behind you—your foot going halfway up toward your butt. Don't reach out too far. That means you are **overstriding** (slowing yourself down by taking steps that are too big).

15 Foot placement: Land on your heel, roll to the front of your foot and push off with the **front of your foot**—not just your toes.

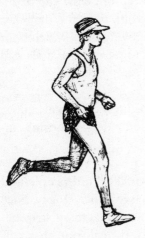

These are basic rules for running form—but one rule supersedes all the others: Do what feels natural.

The perfect **stride** (the overall movement of your legs when running) for you might not be the stride you see on the best runner in your area. Or your **arm carriage** (the way you carry your arms when you run) might not be the same as your training partner's.

Rules of the Road, and Treadmill, and Golf Course and Sidewalk and Trail

In chapter five (see "Surface to Surface," p. 42) I'll cover the running surfaces that you'll encounter training for a **4-hour marathon**. Here, however, I'd like to go over some basic rules for running on them.

ROAD WORK: Always run facing traffic. Keep as far to the side of the road as possible. Slow for intersections and observe traffic lights (but you can run through them as long as there are no cars in sight). Don't play chicken with a car; you will lose. When running with a friend shift to single file when traffic comes along.

TREADMILL: Never get on a moving treadmill. Always make sure it is off and stopped before you step on. Start the treadmill while standing and work up to your pace for that day. Run in the middle to the front of the moving belt. Watch your footfalls on narrow belts because landing on the sides can throw you off balance.

GOLF COURSE: Fine in the early mornings or late evenings. But if it's busy you'll be better off—and safer—choosing another route that day.

SIDEWALKS: Watch for bumps and cracks. And people and cars pulling out of driveways, and pets (see "Nice Doggy, Nice Doug-y," pp. 5–6). When possible run on the grassy strip between the sidewalk and the street. Always call out ahead of you if a large group is in your way.

AIL: Bucolic bliss only interrupted by other runners and bicycles. Run on the right side. Pass on the left side.

TRACK: Run counterclockwise. Faster runners get the inside lanes. If a group ahead of you blocks your path, let them know you're coming and would like them to move out to a slower lane by shouting—but nicely—"please move aside, I'm coming through." Or by shouting "track." It means the same thing—but only to those who know what you're talking about.

NICE DOGGY, NICE DOUG-Y

A runner's two worst enemies on the road are dogs and people.

A simple rule for encountering dogs when running is this: Avoid them at all times if possible. That means if you are running on a street and you see a pack of collarless pit bulls drooling in an alley over a picked-clean corpse, swing very wide or run the other way.

But that also means the same thing when you see a nice old lady walking her terrier on the trail. Give dogs a wide berth at all times. You never know what an animal is going to do—particularly to a moving target.

Likewise, if a dog routinely harasses you on one of your favorite routes, choose another route. Pepper spray or picking up a big stick might only antagonize the dog more. Remember your goal: to train for and run a **4-hour marathon**. Not to rid the world of mean dogs.

The same holds true for Doug. You might hear insults and wolf whistles thrown your way. Or encounter drivers who won't share the road or walkers who won't share the path.

Again, your best weapon is to ignore it or avoid it. And get on with your training. You have better things to do.

In this chapter you learned how to run and where to run. Now let's turn to the fundamental principles of training for a **4-hour marathon,** which in this book refers to any time between 4:00 and 5:00.

t w o

OPRAH, THE MARATHON AND YOU

Speed

Oprah Winfrey ran her first marathon in **4 hours**.

Let me repeat that: Oprah Winfrey ran her first marathon in **4 hours**.

Now no one would ever accuse the talk-show host of being an accomplished athlete. In fact, she was a woman who battled a weight problem (going through a succession of diets) until, lo and behold, she found that running—not just dieting alone—was the key to keeping her weight in check. Of course, you might argue that Oprah had a personal trainer, taking her every step of the way through her marathon training and race. And that, poor old me, I can't afford a personal trainer.

Yes you can. This book **is your personal trainer**, taking you step-by-step to the finish line of a **marathon in 4 hours**.

As I said before, **4 hours** is a **doable goal**. To run a marathon in 4 hours you need to average just a fraction under 9 minutes and 10 seconds per mile. To break it down further, 4 minutes and 35 seconds per half mile, 2 minutes and 17 seconds per quarter mile, or 68 seconds per one-eighth mile.

Take this test: Go to your local track or get on a treadmill at your health club. Now run 220 yards—half a lap or one-eighth of a mile—comfortably.

Chances are you ran that eighth of a mile faster than 68 seconds.

You see, you do have the **speed** to run a **4-hour** marathon. But you probably don't have the **endurance** or **stamina**.

Yet.

You will—in **4 months**.

Unlike speed, which is pretty hard to gain through training, endurance and stamina can be "hot wired" into your body in a matter of months.

First, let's break down our terms.

-------------------------------- 4-HOUR HEROES --------------------------------

Some runners—the "fast guys and girls"—seem to think that if you don't complete a marathon in a certain time, you're not a "real runner," as though you could pick an arbitrary time and say that those runners who can't complete a marathon in, say, three hours aren't "serious runners."

My question with that philosophy has always been: What about the 3:01 marathoners? They run just 2 seconds per mile slower than 3-hour marathoners and yet, they aren't, according to that criteria, "serious runners." But if you concede that point you have to include the 3:02 marathoner because she's only a step behind the 3:01 marathoner . . . and the 3:03

marathoner because she's just a step behind the 3:02 marathoner . . . and so on.

In fact, I agree with 1996 U.S. Olympic Marathoner Keith Brantly, who spoke about 4-hour marathoners a few years ago. He was on a podium about 2 hours after his finish (around 2:15). And he had this answer to a question about how hard it was to run a marathon:

"It's tough. That's why they call it a marathon. But my race is over in about two hours. It's the people who are still out there now [4 hours] that I tip my hat to. They're my heroes."

So be a hero. Start training for a 4-hour marathon.

Endurance: The Long and Winding Road

Endurance means how long you can go without stopping.

My dad, for instance, had very little endurance the first time out the door, running for less than half a mile before he had to stop.

But studies have shown that with the proper endurance workouts and proper rest between those workouts, most runners can improve their endurance dramatically in a matter of weeks. A beginning runner can reasonably increase endurance by about 15 minutes every week.

So. Multiply that 15-minute increase by 16 weeks and a runner who is now going for 30 minutes will be able to run for 4 hours by the end of 4 months of endurance training!

Stamina: Keep the Pace

Being able to run 26.2 miles is only part of your goal. You want to run that 26.2 miles at a 9:10 per-mile pace. That will take **stamina**—the ability to keep going at a steady pace.

Stamina will be a little harder to gain than endurance. But, again, by running one key workout a week, and by getting proper rest, you will see dramatic improvements in your stamina, too.

Take Ernie, for instance. At the beginning of his marathon training he could only hold a 9:10 pace for about 3 miles. Twenty-six miles seemed an eternity to him.

But there is a secret most non-marathoners don't know: The human body is an amazingly adaptable machine. You **stress** it with a five-mile run at a 9-minute pace on Tuesday and by the next Tuesday, if you've given it enough **rest and food**, it will be able to go farther at that same pace. Essentially, what the body is saying to itself is: Hey! I felt a little uncomfortable on Tuesday when you made me run that workout. I'm going to build myself up and get stronger, so that doesn't happen again.

There you have it.

Two goals:

1 To run 26.2 miles: Endurance

2 To run those miles at a 9:10 per-mile pace: Stamina

If you do that, you'll cross the finish line in **4 hours**. That is the goal of this book.

Make no mistake about it, it won't be an **effortless goal**. But it is a **doable goal**.

------------------------------BEFORE YOU BEGIN------------------------------

People beginning the **4 months to a 4-hour marathon** program should have a base level of fitness before they start. You should have been running or doing aerobics or cycling on a regular basis, and be able to do either of those workouts for 45 minutes without stopping.

You might want to take an extra month to get in some **base fitness** before you begin the program. Below is a simple base fitness schedule:

	M	T	W	TH	FRI	SAT	SUN
Week 1	10	off	10	off	15	off	off
Week 2	15	off	15	off	20	off	off
Week 3	20	off	20	off	30	off	off
Week 4	25	off	25	off	40	off	off

NOTE: *Numbers are minutes of easy jogging.*

In this chapter we've gone over endurance, stamina and speed. But before you hit the road, you need to know what to wear.

three

GEAR-ING UP

Shoes

The most important piece of equipment is your **shoes**. That sounds obvious enough but it's worth repeating: The most important piece of equipment is your **shoes**.

Your shoes—not your sports watch or sunglasses or brand-new Gore-Tex rain gear—are what's going to hit the road more than 30,000 times during a 4-hour marathon, and hundreds of thousands of times more than that during training, so you'd better have a good pair. Try this analogy on for size. What would you rather drive to work? A new Mercedes with air, deluxe stereo and . . . two flat tires? Or a no-frills Volkswagen with brand-new tires? See?

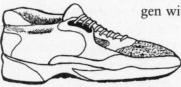

What is a good pair of running shoes? The pair that's right for you. Everyone's foot is different, so the shoe that works for Sam might not work for Sally. Some shoes are made especially for people with wide feet or people with narrow feet. Some are made for heavier runners. Some are made for light-footed runners (the few).

There are several sources of knowledge to tap into when searching for the right shoes. The first would be a **running friend**. Chances are he or she has been through several dozen different pairs, and he or she can give you some words of advice.

Runner's World magazine also puts out a special shoe guide two or three times a year. If you don't subscribe to the magazine you should, and consult those guides. If not, go to the library and look through the back issues until you find those guides.

Other sources include a **good running shoe store**. These are getting easier to find than they were a few years ago. With the second running boom—by the way, by buying this book, you are a part of it—more and more people are running and more and more people who are serious runners are working in shoe stores, and not just in the running meccas of Eugene, Boulder and Gainesville, but in places like Kansas City, Cleveland and Baltimore.

So find a good running shoe store. And find a shoe clerk who runs—hint: It's probably not the guy you see outside the store smoking on his break. Tell that person your running history, what surfaces you run on (see "Surface to Surface," p. 42) and that your goal is to run a 4-hour marathon.

With that information, a shoe clerk who runs should be able to recommend three or four pairs of good training shoes. Try them all on. Jog with them around the store. Make sure you have enough room in the toe box. (That's the area for your toes: Your toes should not be hitting the end of the shoe. If they do that in the store, what's going to happen to your toes on a 20-miler?) The most important thing for each runner, and only you can be the judge of this, is that the shoe feels comfortable.

Good running shoes are those made by major running shoe companies—Nike, Reebok, New Balance, Adidas. Good running shoes are going to cost at least $80 a pair, and sometimes as much as $120 a pair. I know this sounds like a lot, but with shoes—the most important piece of equipment, remember—thou shalt not skimp.

Don't be tempted to save money by getting the $50 bargain-basement models. Those shoes are for the person who is running two miles, two days a week. Try training for a marathon in one of those pairs of shoes and you're asking for trouble. As well as for pain in your feet, shins, knees, back—you get the idea.

If the price is still too high, you can try this—it's a practice that many veteran runners employ, although you're not likely to make any new friends at the local running store.

What you do is go into the store and try on pairs of shoes until you find one you like. Then go home and look through the back pages of *Runner's World* until you've found a **mail-order shoe outlet** and order those shoes through the mail-order company. You can save anywhere from $10 to $30 a pair.

How many pairs should you buy? To train for a **4-hour marathon** I recommend **three pairs**. (That's three pairs of the same model of shoe, a training shoe. Buy the first pair, run in them a few days and if you're happy with them, buy two more pairs.)

You need two pairs to rotate during training. **Rotating shoes** simply means you wear one pair on Monday and the other pair on Tuesday. "It lets them dry out and bounce back," says Ernie. Bouncing back means that the shock absorbers in the midsole (the part between your foot and the sole of the shoe) need time to expand after the compression of running. If they don't get that time, you're running on "crushed" shoes that won't cushion your feet.

So rotate two pairs of training shoes through your training. Then, three weeks before the marathon, put the third pair of shoes into the rotation. You should do five or six short runs in these shoes to break them in. But save the long runs for the other pairs of shoes. Why? Because this third pair is your **race pair**, and you want them to be broken in, not broken down.

Don't be intimidated by the names of some of the shoes: "Gel," "Air" and the like are just what shoe companies are putting into the midsoles of their shoes to, theoretically, help them bounce back faster. Again, the main quality you're looking for in a shoe is your own personal comfort.

What about the **racing flats** you see in stores? Should you buy them for the marathon?

NO. A big NO. Most racing flats—thinner, lighter-weight shoes than trainers—are made to race short distances like 5K and 10K. Though they weigh less and hence feel easier to run in, they won't hold up under the stress of a marathon. (*I have actually seen marathoners with their racing flats split open during the race.*) Or you won't hold up under the stress of the marathon because racing flats don't cushion your feet or stabilize your ankles as much as you need to cover 26 miles. Those runners you see at the starting line in racing flats are invariably **elite** runners, fast men and women blessed with light feet to begin with.

For women, reputable running shoe stores have the shoe selection broken down by sex, and for good reason. Women's feet are different than men's. Women's bodies are different than men's. Women need different running shoes. If you are in a store that doesn't separate shoes by sex, run, don't walk to the nearest store that does so. There are even stores that only carry women's shoes and clothing—Lady Foot Locker, for example.

Finally, **lace locks** can keep laces from coming untied—a great help on wet days. (You should always double-knot your laces on all runs if you don't use lace locks.)

Socks

Socks, like shoes, need to be broken in. That is, don't do the marathon or a long run in a brand-new pair of socks. You're only asking for blisters, even when you use "running socks," socks that have "wicking materials," or "blister-free" socks.

White is the color of choice. (Dark socks bleed.) Cotton or some cotton blend is good. They should fit your foot snugly but not restrict blood flow. Ankle-length socks—often labeled "running socks"—are preferable for two reasons: First, they are long enough so they don't start to "ride" under your foot, which some of the mini-socks can do. Second, they are short enough so that they don't bother you late in the race, unlike tube socks that stretch up to your knees and, late in the race, absorb sweat or rain and hang from each leg like wet cats.

In training you need to have lots of white, cotton ankle socks—say, about eight to ten pairs. Unless you want to be doing laundry every day.

As tempting as it may be to get lazy and let sweaty socks dry out and run in them a day later, don't. Not only do they smell bad, but socks are supposed to be added shock absorbers and a dirty used sock is flat and not a good cushion. It is also full of yesterday's sweat and, maybe, some fungus is growing there too. Dirty socks are an invitation to athlete's foot.

Shorts and Shirts

Summer Gear

Any day over 65 degrees is a summer day for a runner. The simplest summer gear for running—in addition to shoes and socks—consists of running shorts (plus underwear), a T-shirt or singlet (plus running bra for women), and a few accessories. Let's take them one at a time:

Shorts: There are several makes and models. Generally what you're after is a brand name—Nike, Adidas, Reebok, etc.—running short, made of some nylon blend that will wick away sweat and keep you dry. There are two lengths of running shorts: The traditional length which stops about halfway down the thigh, and the newer semi-baggy shorts. They look like basketball shorts and hang almost to the knees. Both are fine for training and racing. But, remember, during the marathon those baggy shorts are going to become wet and the more wet clothing you have hanging from you, the harder it will be to run.

Women have a third option. Close-fitting **briefs** that look like swimsuit bottoms and go by the nickname "bun huggers." These are fine, if you don't feel self-conscious wearing them.

Many runners who are either big in the thigh, bowlegged or both experience chafing on the inside of the thighs. A dab or two of Vaseline before your run can help. Another option is to wear short **mini-tights** (they used to be called tri-shorts because triathletes used them) that cover half the thighs and protect you from that "rubbing problem."

Shorts are one of the easiest pieces of gear to take care of. If you're not fashion conscious you can wear them every day. Just walk into the shower with them after you run, wash them out and hang them to dry. By tomorrow's run they'll be ready to go.

Shirts and **singlets:** A **cotton T-shirt** *is fine up to a point.* That point is roughly what we'll call your "sweat point," i.e., when you're going to finish a run sopping wet. For Ernie, anything over 75 degrees is his sweat point, and he opts instead for a **singlet** made of **Cool Max** material—it wicks the moisture away from the body. Singlets have no sleeves and loop around the shoulders so you don't have the wet patches on your shirt, under your arms, and they also leave free your upper back and part of your chest for added coolness.

Shirtless is also an option for men. When the temperature gets over 80 degrees, you can go shirtless on some of your runs. But watch sunny days so that you don't burn.

Women should wear a **running bra**. There is a wide variety of styles and colors available. Since you'll be running long distance, you'll need a running bra that's made for high-impact activities. Running is different than walking and after a 45-minute run the chest area can become quite sore if there's nothing to support it. Wear a running bra and a T-shirt or a running bra and a singlet (don't worry if it shows outside the singlet: that's the style). Or on hot days, simply a running bra itself.

-------------------------------- HEED THE HEAT --------------------------------

Running in temperatures above 85 degrees, or temperatures above 75 degrees with the humidity over 50 percent, can cause serious problems. If you can, run earlier in the day to avoid severe heat. But if you can't, try to run in as much shade as possible and never be stuck without fluids to drink.

There are three heat-related problems that runners suffer.

Muscle Cramps: Calf and hamstring muscles are where muscle cramps strike most often. Sometimes they are so severe you have to stop running for the day. Other times you can stop, stretch the muscle and then continue. Muscle cramps are caused by dehydration, so drink plenty of fluid before, during and after your runs. You can sweat up to a quart of fluid per half hour and you need to replace that fluid or you will become susceptible to cramps the next time you run in the heat.

Heat Exhaustion: Dizziness, heavy sweating and muscle fatigue that may cause you to actually weave when you run. Heat exhaustion is also caused by dehydration and generally occurs during intense efforts—like races, hard training sessions or long runs. If you start to suffer from any of these symptoms during a run, stop immediately, find a cool place and drink plenty of fluid. Drink much more than you are thirsty for because when your body is severely dehydrated it needs much more fluid than your stomach can hold in one gulp. A good rule of thumb is to drink until you're full and then keep drinking six ounces every ten minutes thereafter—until your urine is clear.

Heatstroke: You stop sweating because you are out of fluid. Your skin is red, hot and dry. And you pass out. Heatstroke is a life-threatening situation and emergency aid involves packing the body in ice to get the core temperature down and calling an ambulance. The best prevention for this is not to tempt fate and train long and hard on oppressively hot days. And especially do not train alone on very hot days.

Learn to Accessorize

If you have sensitive eyes, like many contact lens wearers, **sunglasses** can help on bright days. They not only help you see better but keep you from squinting, which, on a long run, can start to drain you. Many sunglasses are made especially for runners. They are lightweight, padded and really stick on your head. Expect to pay for them too. Brand-name sunglasses can run you more than the cost of your shoes. If you're not concerned so much with brand names, pick some unknown kind after trying them on first. They won't be quite as fashionable as the $180 glasses, but they will serve your purpose. You might also consider getting "croakies" or some other form of sunglasses tether to keep your glasses firmly in place while you run.

A **ball cap** can serve the same purpose as sunglasses, but when it's hot out, remember that most of your heat escapes through the top of your head. Wearing a cap on an 85-degree day is like putting a lid on a pot of boiling water. If you choose a hat on a hot day, try to find a flimsy cotton hat, like the kind cyclists wear. It covers the head, but allows heat to escape. Some runners also like to wear visor-type hats because they shield your eyes but let heat out through the top of your head. But those hats seem to me, at least, to be a little tighter fitting, which can be uncomfortable during a long run.

Sunscreen should be applied during any run longer than half an hour on sunny days. Choose a non-sticky sports brand and apply to the major sun-hitting areas—shoulders, back, ears, back of neck and arms. (Also: If your marathon is on a sunny day apply before your race too. It's amazing how many people get a sunburn during a marathon.)

Lightweight **rain gear** is available for rainy runs on warm days. A light nylon shell can do the trick, but it can also heat up your body faster than you can say, "I wore too many clothes." If it's more than 75 degrees out and raining, who cares if you are going to get wet? Make it a fun run and don't worry about the jacket.

Watch It

The days of runners going around in circles on a track while the coach stands barking out splits from a stopwatch around his neck are the stuff of PBS documentaries. Runners today gauge their own pace with **sports watches**. They come in dozens of brands and do everything from telling the time to taking your pulse.

You can buy a deluxe model. But all you really need is a model that shifts to **stopwatch mode** so you can get a running time on your runs and **splits** (sections of your run, say, mile splits on a 10-mile run). Just make sure that the buttons are easy to press, *and* that the readout is big enough to see while you are running. It's not the same as pressing the buttons and looking at the readout while standing still in the bright lights of the store.

ERNIE'S TIP: DRESS FOR SUCCESS

Whatever your running outfit—warm or cold weather—try to dress in neat, clean, coordinated clothing. "It helps promote a good self-image and confidence," says Ernie. "And confidence means a lot when you're running a marathon because the race, you'll find out in the later miles, is really about how you feel about yourself."

Cold Comfort

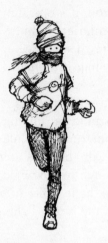

Any running days cooler than 50 degrees are **cold weather days**. On the **in-between days**—50–65 degrees—you can dress in shorts and a long-sleeved shirt or sweatshirt (depending on how you handle the cold). But once the mercury dips into the 40s, you need to do some serious thinking about what to wear.

Let's start from the top: **Hats** are your number-one weapon against the cold. On cold days, think of your body as a teakettle when you run. The heat that you generate boils over and comes out the top—your head—unless you have something on it—a hat.

A **baseball cap** can do the trick for days in the high 40s, but on any other days you'll need a **knit cap** or a **wool ski cap**. Try several on. Make sure they cover your ears (some styles have extra lining around the ears) but don't "droop" too far down. Also make sure they feel comfortable. This hat will see you through long runs and maybe even your marathon (if that day is cold), so make sure it's a snug, comfortable fit.

For days colder than 20 degrees, you might want to wear a **ski mask** that covers your face and protects your cheeks from frostbite. Or slather some **petroleum jelly** on your face. It's a good insulator.

Sunglasses, of course, will come in handy on bright, snow-covered days.

For the torso, your best bet is to **dress in layers**. This strategy is preferable for two reasons: Layers keep you warmer, and you can always strip off your top layer if you get too warm.

THE CARDINAL RULE: BE A BIRD OF MANY FEATHERS

The cardinal rule of running in the cold is to *over-dress rather than underdress*. If you underdress and you get 5 miles into your 18-miler and the wind kicks up, you're suddenly like some arctic explorer who is 85 miles from nowhere and out of food and canned heat.

Three layers should be enough for the coldest days. Your bottom layer should consist of a **long-sleeved, lycra-type shirt**. The fabric will wick away moisture from your body, keeping you dry. The second layer is your insulation: A **cotton turtleneck or a heavier sweatshirt** can do the trick. Your third layer is some kind of shell to protect you from the wind and keep in the heat. **Nylon windbreakers** are good for most days. On days colder than 20 degrees you might want to keep a **Gore-Tex top** handy. Gore-Tex lets moisture out and keeps heat in.

Experiment on your short runs with the clothes you feel comfortable with so you will be ready and comfortable on any long runs in cold weather.

Gloves are another essential item for cold weather days. Lightweight cotton **painter's gloves** are fine for days in the 40s. But on days when the temperature is below that you should have snugger **polypropylene** models. Gloves are something you should also take along with you on all cold weather running days—even borderline warm days because you never know when the wind will kick up. Gloves are easy to take on and off. Just tuck them inside your jacket pockets or fold them into the waistband of your shorts or sweatpants. Then put them back on if your hands get cold.

From the waist down you have several options. Some

people might be able to wear shorts in 40-degree weather. Others can don **tights**. These come in three models: nylon tights, looser-fitting stirrup-type tights (Sport Hill puts out a nice selection of these) and thick, polypropylene tights.

You can wear your regular running shorts underneath your snug tights (if they don't "bunch" too much) or a non-binding pair of underwear. Stirrup tights, a favorite of Ernie's, are loose enough so that regular running shorts won't cause a problem. Some people wear running shorts over their nylon tights. This adds an extra layer of warmth and modesty.

On days colder than 30 degrees, men should consider an extra layer: **Polypropylene** briefs, then running shorts, then stirrup tights.

Another option for cold days is traditional **warmup pants**—long, nylon-shelled pants that open with zippers near your feet. On days colder than 20 degrees you can wear tights beneath the warmups.

The same **socks** you wear for warm days will work on cold days. Just remember to pick clean ones, since dirty, used ones will have used up most of their absorption, and wet feet in 20-degree weather soon become cold feet. One pair is all you need. Two pairs might cause blisters and will cramp your feet in your shoes.

The same **shoes** you train in will be fine for cold weather days. Just remember to keep running! As long as you're running you'll generate heat. So don't end your run 1 mile from your house or car and walk a **cool-down** (5 or 10 minutes after your run when you let your body relax by walking). You can always cool down in the gym or den.

A final note: What you wear depends on the weather but it also depends on what workout you're going to do that day. If Ernie is out the door to do a long run in 40-degree weather he will be bundled up in three layers and tights. But if on that same day he is going to do a 6-mile tempo run on a trail, he'll wear just two layers and maybe even shorts. The reasoning: "I generate more heat when I'm doing a tempo run," he says. "I know I'll be warmer, so I don't dress as heavily. I just make sure I don't end the workout too far away from dry clothes or a hot shower."

COLD CONDITIONS

Here are the rules for running in cold weather:

1. Dress in layers.

2. Don't be afraid to overdress (you can always remove clothing).

3. Watch out for icy sidewalks and streets. If you can run on a path, take the path.

4. Run into the wind on the way out and with the wind on the way back.

5. Wear a hat and gloves to curb heat loss.

6. Don't stand outside after your run.

7. Change into dry clothes as quickly as possible.

8. Drink during long runs: You sweat just as much on cold days, so replace those fluids.

9. Spend more time warming up, especially for a fast run.

10. Run with a friend.

11. Wear sunglasses on bright, snowy days.

12. Heed the first sign of frostbite: The skin appears blue. Immediate treatment is keeping the

area warm by dunking it in warm water or wrapping it in extra clothing.

13. If it's colder than 10, 15 or 20 degrees (your choice) run inside.

14. Drink hot liquids to warm the body after your run.

Dressing for Success

Here is a shorthand reminder of what to wear when you run in particular temperatures.

80s: shorts, singlet.

70s: shorts, singlet.

60s: shorts, T-shirt or long-sleeved T-shirt.

50s: shorts or tights, long-sleeved T-shirt or sweatshirt.

40s: shorts or tights, two layers (long-sleeved, T-shirt over), hat, gloves.

30s: tights or pants, three layers (Nylon top), hat, gloves.

20s: tights or pants, three layers (Gore-Tex top), hat, gloves.

10s: tights and pants, three layers (Gore-Tex top), hat, gloves.

Note: We will cover marathon-day clothing in chapter eight.

Now that you know what to wear—in every conceivable type weather—let's turn to what to eat.

four

CARBO-NATED

Fuel for the Marathon

While training for a **4-hour marathon**, keep this analogy in mind: Your body is a car. Your leg muscles are the fuel tanks. When you run, you burn that fuel. After you run, you need to fill the tanks back up again, or next time you'll be running on empty.

The only fuel that works is: **carbohydrates**.

This, of course, is an oversimplification. You need fat and protein too. But the primary fuel source for all your running is carbohydrates, "carbs" for short—breads, pastas, beans, sugars, etc.

Your nutritional goal, then, while training for a 4-hour marathon, is to keep the carbohydrate tanks filled. This means doing two things: eating a high-carbohydrate diet (but a diet that includes fat and protein too), and refueling your muscles immediately after intense efforts,

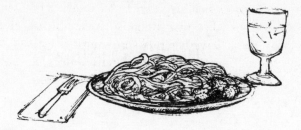

such as Wednesday's turnover and tempo runs, and Saturday's long runs (see next chapter).

A high-carbohydrate diet does not mean stuffing yourself with carbohydrates all day long. During your training, a good practice to keep the tanks full is to make one meal a day your carb-refueling meal. Say to yourself: Monday's breakfast is going to fill the tanks (then have a stack of pancakes). Or: Tuesday's lunch is going to fill the tanks (then have a pasta salad). Or: Wednesday's dinner is going to fill the tanks (then have beans and rice). The other meals you will eat sensibly, getting some carbohydrates but not forcing pasta down your throat like it was medicine for a child: You simply don't need that much, can't store that much, or can't tolerate that much. Going hog wild on fruit can cause diarrhea. Too many bagels and you get the opposite effect.

Also, be sure to eat some **fat and protein** each day—say, a piece of cheese on your turkey sandwich. The fat and protein will help keep your hunger on even keel (an all-carbohydrate diet can make you crave more food soon after eating because carbohydrates burn quickly). Fats and proteins also help in your training. **Fat** helps fuel your long runs. **Protein** helps re-build leg muscles after hard workouts and aids in energy transport during runs. You need all three to have a balance in your diet and get the best performance while you run.

After your Wednesday and Saturday workouts, eat some carbohydrates—say, a bagel or a banana—or drink a carbohydrate-replacement fluid, *immediately* after you finish. This will help refuel your muscles when they are **most susceptible to refueling**.

Think of it this way: The tanks in your legs are wide open for about 20 minutes following an intense effort. So take full advantage of this. This is *vital* to help tired legs recover in time for your next important workout.

FAD DIETS

Cut carbs. Load up on protein. Only drink fluids.

A word about fad diets while you are training for your 4-hour marathon: DON'T.

You want to keep energy levels as high and consistent as possible—otherwise you'll slow recovery and feel too worn out to train—and the way you do that is by eating a healthy, balanced runner's diet.

The Two Most Important Meals of the Week: Wednesday Dinner and Saturday Brunch

WEDNESDAY DINNER: Following the **4 months to a 4-hour marathon** schedule you will be running an intense workout almost every Wednesday evening.

Immediately after this workout, get some carbs in you in the form of a light snack or an energy drink. Then, within the next hour, sit down to a high-carbohydrate meal: pasta, or beans and rice, or baked potatoes and broccoli.

SATURDAY BRUNCH: A weekly long run on Saturday morning is a keystone in training for a **4-hour marathon**.

Immediately after your long run, get some carbs in you in the form of food or an energy drink. Then, within an hour, sit down to a high-carbohydrate brunch: pancakes, waffles or oatmeal.

ERNIE'S TIP

"Make these meals special," he says. "Do these workouts with friends who are also training for a 4-hour marathon. And then meet afterward at a restaurant or someone's house. On Saturday-morning long runs, for instance, I run with friends and then we meet at a restaurant where lots of runners hang out."

Marathon Week Meal Schedule

What you eat the week before a marathon is vital to run a 4-hour marathon. You will have been cutting back on your running drastically, so you might be tempted to cut back on your eating too—don't. This is the time you **actually fuel** your body for the 4-hour marathon.

But those last seven days come with some caveats: Don't overeat. And don't eat the wrong stuff—fatty foods, like deep-dish pizzas and cheese omelettes. You might actually crave this stuff—due to a mixture of nerves, your body's reaction to not running so much and getting sick and tired of spaghetti every night. Therefore, I've outlined a seven-day nutritional schedule for that last week before your 4-hour marathon. It serves a dual purpose: to store the carbohydrates and to keep your taste buds happy.

MONDAY
    Breakfast: Cereal with skim milk, banana, glass of orange juice.
    Lunch: Turkey sandwich, and water or fruit juice.
    Dinner: Pasta with red sauce or a little meat sauce, skim milk, salad.

TUESDAY
    Breakfast: Bagel(s), orange juice.
    Lunch: Cold pasta salad with chicken.
    Dinner: Red beans and rice.

WEDNESDAY
    Breakfast: Pancakes with bananas.
    Lunch: Grilled chicken sandwich.
    Dinner: Chinese food with extra rice (no MSG).

THURSDAY
  Breakfast: Cereal with bananas, orange juice.
  Lunch: Tuna fish sandwich, pretzels.
  Dinner: Pasta with red sauce (and ground turkey), salad.

FRIDAY
  Breakfast: Pancakes with bananas, orange juice.
  Lunch: Cold pasta with chicken.
  Dinner: Red beans and rice, salad.

SATURDAY (DAY BEFORE THE MARATHON)
  Breakfast: Cereal with bananas.
  Lunch: Grilled chicken sandwich.
  Dinner: Your choice, but remember to eat early. Most
  marathons start at eight or nine in the morning, so if you
  eat a late dinner the night before, you not only disrupt
  what little rest you'll get, but you also might spend more
  time in the bathroom before the race than you counted on.

Pre-Race Meal

Two to three hours before the marathon you should eat a
light carbohydrate meal. This meal is the one you've been eating before Saturday morning long runs (example: a toasted
bagel and a half a banana). The purpose of this meal is **not** to
fuel you through the marathon (the glycogen stored in your
muscles and liver plus body fat will provide your fuel). You
need to eat something beforehand to get you to the starting
line **not** feeling hungry or light-headed because of low blood
sugar. And therefore, ready to run.

Katie Don't Bar the Door: Energy Bars

Compact and packed with calories and vitamins and electrolytes, energy bars do not bruise or squish like fruit or a

peanut butter sandwich. Which makes them perfect food for 4-hour marathoners.

All the bars listed below can be consumed post-workout or post-race, but you'll need to eat and learn before you pick which bar is best to be consumed during the race. (Hint: Cut into bite-sized pieces and pop one in your mouth every five miles or so.)

That said, here is a quick review of the top four energy bars:

Power Bar: The original energy bar still has a lot going for it. Vitamins and minerals and electrolytes (the new Protein Plus Power Bar has 22 grams of protein). Yet it is also chewy and contains some fiber, which could lead to an upset stomach during your marathon.

Cliff Bar: Some fat to go along with vitamins, minerals and electrolytes, which makes this bar more desirable during training. For marathons, 9 grams of fiber could be too much for your stomach.

Zone Perfect: Saturated fat but easy to chew and digest because of its low fiber content. Smaller size. Recommended for marathons.

Balance Gold: Like the Zone Perfect in size and content. Recommended for marathons.

Fuel for the Wall

If you haven't heard the term yet, let me introduce you to "The Wall." It sits out there on the marathon course, somewhere between 16 and 22 miles. Once you hit it, you'll know it—it's accompanied by a feeling of total exhaustion: mental and physical, due to low blood sugar and your body running out of glycogen. After your first marathon, you will never forget it.

The Wall is the bogeyman for marathoners. But once you learn how to deal with it, the mystique is taken away—sort of like drawing back the curtain to reveal that the Great and All-Powerful Oz is just a man working some levers.

First off, you need to eat the week before the marathon. Check.

Second, you need to eat the morning of the marathon. Check.

And finally, you need to get some carbohydrates in you **during the marathon.** Carbs can come in several forms: energy drinks at the water stops, energy bars that you've cut up and stuffed in your shorts or fanny pack . . . hard candies, cookies in a bag, gels, Fig Newtons . . . whatever you have practiced with during your long runs.

The purpose of **fueling** yourself during the marathon is to avoid low blood sugar—the first indication that the Wall is looming—and to refuel your muscles with carbohydrates.

For 4-hour marathoners that means taking along at least four doses—one every hour or so—to keep you feeling alert and ahead of the Wall.

The **one-hour rule** is not a constant. If you start feeling light-headed before that, by all means pop a hard candy into your mouth. The point is, you don't want to get to the point where you're feeling so light-headed that you desperately need to eat. By that point you've already tempted fate. So stay ahead of the feeling and you'll do fine.

The final way to prevent the Wall is to drink lots of water during your race. Dehydration is another way to hit the Wall. The best insurance is to drink like you were voting for the Mayor of Chicago in the 1920s: early and often.

Marathon Hydration

Gatorade. Powerade. Gatorade Endurance Formula. Powerade Option.

There are enough energy/replacement drink options to fill

a grocery store shelf, probably two shelves. Many known brands like Gatorade and Powerade now make "upgrade" versions like Gatorade's Endurance Formula, which is a thicker more concentrated version of regular Gatorade (it has more sodium and potassium but might be harder on your stomach) or low-cal versions, like Powerade Option.

Which drink, then, should you choose in training for your 4-hour marathon? The answer is simple: the drink that will be passed out to you at water stops during your marathon.

You can find the exact drink by contacting the marathon or its website. Even go so far as to inquire about the flavor—there is a big difference sometimes between lemon-lime and orange and some of the newer flavors, and you need to have your tongue, palate and stomach accustomed to it all before the big day.

Also find out if the drink will be powdered (there is a difference) and, if it is, try mixing that in your water bottles during long runs in the weeks and months before race day.

Coffee? Tea? Genessee?

Cut out caffeine—coffee, tea, most soft drinks—three days before the marathon. Likewise with alcohol, preferably the week before or more. Caffeine and alcohol are diuretics—they suck water from your body. Plus, alcohol can interfere with the storage of glycogen in your liver, the fuel that will carry you through the marathon.

(You might have heard stories about Olympic runners quaffing beers the day before their races. Those stories might be true. But what is also true is that they were Olympic runners. Their metabolisms are different from ours.)

Water, Water, Everywhere

You should be drinking water all the time. But in the days leading up to the race, water is especially important. A good rule is to drink until your urine is clear. Then drink 6 ounces every hour.

Sports drinks can be used too—but use them sparingly. They contain lots of sugars—good for the marathon itself and for refueling. But the danger with sports drinks is that you can easily overdo it. You drink way too much and come to marathon day sugar-saturated and feeling bloated.

We know how to supercharge ourselves with food and drink. Now let's get out there and train.

five

THE HIGH FIVE: WORKOUTS TO RUN A 4-HOUR MARATHON

You've got 4 months to train for a 4-hour marathon. That's 16 weeks—102 days. Plus race week.

Four months is the optimal amount of time to train for a marathon, for two reasons. First, you **can** get ready for a marathon in that time. Second, it's a short enough span—shorter than, say, a six-month or one-year buildup program—so that you don't get **burned out** on the training before the race begins. You want to enter the race with fresh, expectant legs, not legs that were worn out two months ago, which is a major mistake made by many people training for a marathon.

Training for a 4-hour marathon will be tough. Your nonrunning friends will look at you sideways when you say you have to go home and be in bed by 10 o'clock (you will need extra sleep, at least 30 minutes to an hour or two more than normal on most nights). And you will pass on dessert (sugar is not a good fuel) and other activities because you just don't have the energy for it all.

Get used to saying this sentence now: "I'm training for a 4-hour marathon."

Again: "I'm training for a 4-hour marathon." Believe me, you will use this sentence to explain yourself several times a week.

Okay, let's start training.

Types of Workouts

The **4 months to a 4-hour marathon** training program is simple. Each day you will be doing one of just five workouts. That's right, you need just five types of workouts to get in shape for a 4-hour marathon. Let's look at them one at a time.

Workout #1: Long Runs

The major goal of any marathoner is "conquering the distance." The way you make sure you do this is by long runs.

The distance of your long run is relative. (It depends on what part of the training program you're in.) When you first start the program it will be 7 miles. By the time you finish the program it will be 24 miles. When I say "long run," I mean any run that's geared specifically toward increasing your endurance. Long runs are run slower than 4-hour marathon pace (9 minutes and 10 seconds per mile), at least 90 seconds to 2 minutes per mile slower than race pace. So your window is 10:40 to 11:10.

The reason why you run long runs slowly is that in order to build endurance **you do not need to run fast.** So why risk injury or burnout by running at race pace?

AEROBIC ENEMY NUMBER ONE:
FAST LONG RUNS

Fast long runs are the number-one training mistake for beginning marathoners. They want to run their 16-to-20-milers at marathon pace. And all that does for them is make the workout a marathon in itself. That makes them too tired to run the next week. Or worse, injured.

Therefore, **the 4 months to a 4-hour marathon** program has you running your long runs 90 seconds to 2 minutes slower per mile than marathon race pace.

This does four things: It gives you endurance. Remember, endurance does not depend on speed. It makes you tired but not so worn out that you can't run again that week. It keeps you from being injured. And it keeps you hungry. The marathon will be a "racing experience" that you haven't done four or five times in training.

LONG-RUN WORKOUT: Run 7 to 24 miles at a 10:40 to 11:10 pace. (The distance will depend on what week of training you are into.) The goal is to keep running. If you need to, stop and walk occasionally, but don't make this a habit late in your long run. You will be tired, and once you start walking it will take more effort to start running again. Oprah ran every step of her marathon; you can too.

Long-Run Tips

1 Start slow, finish slow: Long runs are not races. Run them by yourself or with friends who are also training for

a 4-hour marathon. The goal is to finish the run at the same pace you started.

2 Eat and drink: Practice taking fluids and fuel during your long runs in preparation for the marathon. Fluids should come every 2–3 miles. (Drink early and drink often. If you're thirsty, it's almost too late.) Place "squeeze bottles" out on the course.

Also, fuel yourself with fluids (energy drinks are packed with carbohydrates) or practice with energy gels (a carbohydrate gel) or some sort of solid fuel (cut-up energy bars, such as a PR Bar; small candies; Fig Newtons). Mix and match on your long runs until you find what works best for you and your stomach. (The best way to carry your fuel is in a **fanny pack**.)

And don't start a long run hungry. Eat a light carbohydrate-rich meal or snack 1 to 2 hours before your run. That means if you are doing your long run at 8 o'-clock Saturday morning, set your alarm clock for 6:30 A.M., have, say, a bagel and a banana and drink lots of water—the best fluid before any long run. This ensures that you don't start your long run light-headed because of low blood sugar or dehydration.

3 Run flat out: Running 16 to 24 miles will be workout enough without having to go up and down too. (Downhill running actually does more damage to your legs than running uphill). Unless your target marathon undulates like a belly dancer's hips (and if you're smart you'll pick a flat marathon for your first time. See chapter ten, "Recommended Marathons for 4-Hour Marathoners," pp. 107–110), we suggest you stick to flat courses in your training runs.

4 Out and back: That means a course that has a turnaround. For instance, to do a 14-mile-long run you would run **out** 7 miles, then **back** to where you started from. **Out and back** courses are easy to measure, and less mentally taxing than running, say, seven times around a **2-mile loop course**.

5 Surface to surface: Choose a soft surface for your long runs (see "Surface to Surface," p. 42). Your legs will thank you the next day and you'll recover more quickly and be ready for the next hard workout.

Warning: Most marathons are run on city streets (concrete and asphalt). So plan to do recovery runs, or parts of your long runs in the weeks prior to the marathon, on pavement. Training all the time on the soft surface of a park trail, then jumping onto the concrete on marathon day, will be a jarring shock to your body. You will be sore before you've run 18 miles and be tempted to drop out.

ERNIE'S LONG-RUN TIP

"Run a route that people use," he says. "You are going to be out there for several hours and if you choose a deserted road, that will make the run all the more difficult psychologically. So choose a well-traveled trail or map out a course that goes through busy parks. Also, you need to practice drinking. It's not as easy as it looks and sometimes I still find it difficult. So I use long runs to practice this marathon technique as well, setting water bottles out at certain mileage points and stopping and drinking." (See also "Boys & Girls," pp. 77–79.)

SURFACE TO SURFACE:
RANKING THE TRAINING VENUES

The best training surface is one that "gives" when your foot lands on it, transferring some of the shock into the surface, rather than up into your knees, hips and back, but doesn't give too much so that you sink into it, causing you to pull your foot out, like it was caught in a vat of molasses. A good running surface is also smooth—no holes or bumps or ruts that will disrupt your stride or twist an ankle.

My order of preference for running surfaces:

1. Well-tended park trails made of dirt or crushed stone over dirt. These have maximum give and good footing. Many of the new Rails to Trails paths are like this.

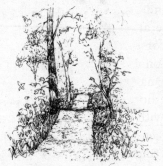

2. Grass. Excellent give, but grass "fields" can be uneven. Golf courses are ideal—but can you run a 20-mile long run around a golf course? Fore!

3. Track: Lots of give but lots of boredom. A 20-miler on the track (80 laps!) will force you to quit your training program faster than any injury.

4. Treadmill. Lots of give, good for recovery days, but monotonous for long runs.

5. Asphalt roads: Will simulate race conditions. Some give and widely available. Don't run on it every day.

6. Concrete: Poison to the legs. Avoid if possible on all long runs. You are most likely going to tramp on some concrete during your marathon. That will be enough.

Workout #2: Quarter-Mile Repeats

This workout is geared toward **turnover**, moving your legs around faster than normal and getting your legs ready to **cruise** at **marathon pace**. An outdoor track is the preferable site for quarter-mile repeats. Or you can measure a quarter mile on a flat trail or side street.

Quarter-mile repeats will be run much faster than marathon pace. You will do six to sixteen repeats in one workout with 2 minutes of rest in between. Quarter-mile repeats will get your legs used to going around faster than on your long runs—but for not nearly so long a distance or time. Sixteen quarter-mile repeats equals four miles of running.

THE WORKOUT: Six to sixteen x 400 meters in 2 minutes with a 2-minute rest in between each. A quarter mile—or 400 meters—is one lap around the track.

Warm up by jogging for 10 minutes. Stretch. Then start your repeats by clicking your sports watch. Don't start out too fast. Your speed should stay constant. Monitor your speed every 200 meters (1 minute) to make sure. After a while you'll get used to the pace and you won't have to check your watch every 200 meters. (Try for a 4-minute pace—that's 2 minutes per quarter mile—but if you can't handle that right away, try for 2:05 to 2:15.)

FRIENDS IN SPEED

Speed workouts are one of the best times to run with a friend who is also training for a marathon. Knowing a friend is meeting you at the track Wednesday night for 10 times a quarter mile will make it a lot harder to blow off. Plus, you can encourage each other and take turns leading each repeat. And, most important, you can keep each other from running too fast, which is pretty easy to do when it's just you and the stopwatch.

You can also agree to meet this friend, or preferably a group of friends, for the Saturday morning long runs. Three- and four-hour runs are tough enough when it's only you and the sparrows. You'll be surprised how much easier those workouts become when you have someone to share them with.

If you don't already know someone who is training for a marathon, you may want to find someone on your level to train with. To find a training partner, be on the lookout at your local trail or path. Talk up your training with other runners until you find someone with similar goals. Some running shoe stores also provide bulletin boards for training partners, as do local running clubs. Find them and use them.

Many running clubs also organize group workouts—speed runs one night a week and Saturday morning long runs. Call and find out when and where they are, and you're bound to find several runners training at your level.

At the end of each repeat, stop your watch and look at your time. If you ran 2 minutes, good job. If you ran 1:50, you've gone too fast. (This is a workout of **accumulation**: The goal is to run your last 400 meters as smoothly as your first.) Start your watch again and walk or jog back and forth by the starting line (you might want to sip water from your water bottle) while you **recover** for 2 minutes. When 2 minutes are just about up, reset your watch and toe the line. You're off.

You should tackle this workout in fours. That is, if you have twelve or sixteen x 400 meter repeats to do, do four in a set. Then walk/jog for five minutes before your next set.

After the last repeat, jog for 10 minutes to cool down. Then your workout is complete.

Quarter-Mile Repeat Tips

1 "This is a fast workout," says Ernie. "But it doesn't tax the lungs as much as it teaches the legs. At first, this workout might seem difficult. But give the body time to adapt. After two or three weeks, you'll be in the swing of things."

2 Run with a friend who is also training for a 4-hour marathon. Take turns leading each quarter-mile repeat. But resist the urge to race. Your race is the marathon, remember.

3 This is a fun day. You'll find that quarter-mile repeats, especially with a group of friends, can be one of the most rewarding workouts. Psych yourself up for this workout hours ahead of time by imagining yourself running fast while you are still seated at your desk.

4 Eat a carbohydrate snack—cookies, banana, energy bar, etc.—or have an energy drink immediately after finishing, to replenish carbohydrates. Also, make sure you have a carbohydrate snack one to two hours **before** this workout.

This ensures that you're feeling up to the challenge and won't drop out after, say, four quarter-mile repeats when the workout is scheduled for eight.

Workout #3: Tempo Runs

Tempo runs help you make marathon-race pace—which will be between 9:00 and 9:05 per mile—feel easy (see "Marathon-Race Pace," p. 60). Your tempo runs, then, will be done between 8:45 and 8:50 per mile (the faster pace will make your marathon pace feel easier), and last between 4 and 8 miles.

Tempo runs are **stamina workouts**. You combine the **turnover** you have learned from quarter-mile repeats and the **endurance** you have gained from your long runs.

THE TEMPO WORKOUT: Warm up with 10 minutes of jogging. Stretch. Run 4 to 8 miles at tempo pace. Cool down with 10 minutes of jogging.

Tempo Tips

1 Concentration is the key. Your goal is to hold this pace for the entire workout. The pace should feel a tad uncomfortable at times, but you are going to run slower than this during the marathon. That's the secret: Tempo runs will teach your body to make marathon pace feel easy!

2 Run with friends who are training for a 4-hour marathon, but don't race.

3 Start slower rather than faster. Busting out the first mile in 8:20 (and there will be this temptation because your

turnover from quarter-mile repeats has taught your legs to do this) might feel good, but it will leave you gasping at the end of 8 miles.

4 Run on a good surface (see "Surface to Surface," p. 42).

5 Have a carbohydrate snack one to two hours before.

6 Eat a carbohydrate snack or drink an energy-replacement drink immediately after finishing.

Workout #4: Recovery Runs/Workouts

Recovery workouts will consist of easy jogging or cross training (cycle, swim, walk or go easy on the stair climber). Recovery is more essential to training for a **4-hour** marathon than any of the above workouts. You might ask: How can jogging 20 minutes be as important as doing a 20-mile run? The answer is simple: In order for your body to become stronger—to "get fit" enough to run a **4-hour** marathon— two things need to happen. One is that you **stress** the body through the three workouts above. The other is that you give the body time to recover and grow stronger. It's pretty easy to see that all work and no recovery can make Jack or Jill a worn-out, injured (a tired body is more susceptible to in- juries), runny-nosed (a tired body is more susceptible to colds) boy or girl.

Therefore *I cannot stress enough the importance* of recov- ery days in your training schedule. If you skip them, you'll end up skipping the marathon.

THE WORKOUT: Jog—1 minute per mile slower than long- run pace—no more than 30 minutes. Or do the equivalent through **cross training**.

Cross training means "cross over" to an alternate workout. It's a good tool for recovery days because it not only lets your body recover from the stress of running, but your mind as well—you're doing something new. Acceptable cross training workouts are cycling or swimming or light aerobics (basketball or racquetball can lead to injuries; the stair stepper is too much like running, so your legs don't get much of a rest). This should be a very easy workout. If you get 10 minutes into your workout and feel exhausted, **slow down even more**. Or consider taking the day off completely.

Recovery Workout Tips

1 Run on soft surfaces.

2 Limit to 20–30 minutes: The purpose of this workout is **recovery**. You *will not* help yourself by going longer.

3 Use your watch to make sure you are going slow enough. A key rule for recovery workouts is: you can't go too slow. Repeat that to yourself as you run or cycle.

Workout #5: Rest Day

The training puzzle is not complete without rest days—days when you do no running or cross training at all, days when you purposely are lazy. Rest days come at least once every six days, and like recovery workouts are **key to training** for a **4-hour marathon**.

THE WORKOUT: No running or cross training at all.

Rest Day Tips

1 Sleep in. Most rest days come on Sundays, so if you can, use that time to get extra sleep. Or sneak a nap in the afternoon.

2 Eat. The temptation will be to cut back on food because you're not running this day. Don't give into it! Instead eat carbohydrate-rich foods to replenish your stores. Just don't overeat.

3 Be like Fido: Sit! Sit!

4 Plan something fun but not taxing, so you won't be tempted to "sneak out" for a run. Go to a movie or play. Read a good book. Go out to eat. Go to a ball game. Spend "quality time" with your wife and kids, husband and kids, girlfriend or boyfriend. They've missed you with all the training you've been doing.

In this chapter you learned the individual types of workouts you'll do in training for a 4-hour marathon. Now you'll find out how they fit in the overall training strategy.

THE THREE PHASES

The **4 months to a 4-hour marathon** training program is broken down into three training phases.

1 The first phase, **the endurance phase,** lasts eight weeks and focuses on endurance with a secondary emphasis on leg turnover.

2 The second phase, **the stamina phase,** lasts six weeks and focuses on stamina, while continuing to increase endurance.

3 The final phase, **the taper phase,** lasts two weeks and focuses on resting the body before marathon week.

Endurance

A) The key workout is the weekly long run, starting at a 7-mile-long run and ending at a 19-mile-long run (during the stamina phase, you will work up to a 24-mile-long run before the marathon).

B) The supplemental workout will be repeat quarter miles, starting at six times a quarter mile and ending at sixteen times a quarter mile.

C) There will be three or four days for recovery jogging or cross training.

D) You'll also have one or two days of total rest.

A typical week in the *endurance phase*

Monday—Jog 40 minutes.
Tuesday—Cross train 30 minutes.
Wednesday—Run twelve x 400 at 2:10 pace.
Thursday—Cross train 30 minutes or rest.
Friday—Jog 30 minutes.
Saturday—Long run of 10–15 miles.
Sunday—Rest day.

Stamina

A) The key workout is the **long run,** which will peak at 24 miles.

B) The supplemental workout is the **tempo run** of 6 to 10 miles.

C) There will be three or four days for recovery jogging/ cross training.

D) You'll have one or two days of rest.

A typical week in the *stamina phase*

Monday—Jog 40 minutes.
Tuesday—Cross train 30 minutes.

Wednesday—8-mile tempo run at 8:50 pace.
Thursday—Cross train 30 minutes or rest.
Friday—Jog 30 minutes or rest.
Saturday—Long run of 21 miles.
Sunday—Rest.

Taper

A) The key workout is easy jogging or cross training three days a week.
B) The supplemental workout is a **10-mile-long run** at long-run pace.
C) Another supplemental workout is a **marathon-pace run** at 9:00 pace.
D) You'll have two to three rest days.

A typical week in the *taper phase*

Monday—Jog 40 minutes.
Tuesday—Cross train 30 minutes.
Wednesday—Rest.
Thursday—**marathon pace** 6-mile run.
Friday—Cross train 30 minutes or rest.
Saturday—**10-mile-long run**.
Sunday—Rest.

WEEKLY MILEAGE VERSUS KEY WORKOUTS?

Weekly mileage—the number of miles you run each week—is a catch phrase among many marathoners. It's a supposed badge of honor that, more often than not, becomes a cross to bear.

You see, when you become a slave to the weekly mileage chart—forcing yourself to run 40 miles this week, and 45 the next week, and 50 miles the week after that and . . . so on, you neglect rest and make yourself susceptible to injuries.

So if you find yourself in a conversation with a weekly mileage junkie, remind yourself that it's high-quality key workouts (long runs, tempo runs, turnover runs and . . . rest and recovery days) that will get you across the finish line in **4 hours**, not the number you pencil in on your training diary every seven days.

THE KEY WORKOUT TO RUNNING A 4-HOUR MARATHON

Marathon lore tells us that the most important workout in your training schedule is your **long run**. The **long run** best simulates the actual marathon and increases your endurance, so that you can cover 26.2 miles. But the **long run** really *isn't* your key workout to running a **4-hour marathon**.

"What?!" you might say. "How can that be? You just said the long run was the most important."

Let me explain: The fast guys, the two-hour-and-fifteen-minute marathoners, do long runs that rarely last marathon 2 hours. On the next day their legs are ready to go an "easy" 8 to 12 miles or so. But **4-hour** marathoners will be doing long runs in twice that amount of time. That's a lot of running and a lot of pounding on your legs.

Therefore, the **key workout** in training for a **4-hour marathon** is the **rest day after your long run**. This is when your body recovers and grows stronger. The workout is not as easy as it sounds. The day after your long run you will be tired but pumped. Hey! I did 18 miles yesterday, I want to go down to the track and tell all the guys about it while I do a 7-mile run!

No. Go directly to the couch and prop up your feet, turn on the tube or open a good book. Remember the credo: **Training is also resting.** Better to rest now than at the 21-mile mark of your marathon because your body is tired or injured.

And remember your goal: to run a 4-hour marathon. Not to impress your friends with your training!

Rest or Run?

Here's a final word on the value of rest in your training schedule. A good rule of thumb is this: Skip a hard workout but never a rest day. Talking to a group of marathoners a few years back, Boston Marathon champ Bill Rodgers said that the most important piece of advice in marathon running he'd ever received was this:

Get to the starting line healthy.

And you can only do that if you rest often and wisely.

In this chapter you learned how the certain workouts become important during certain parts of training. Now let's look at the training schedules themselves. Let's see exactly what we will be running each day for 4 months.

s e v e n

TRAINING SCHEDULES: 16 WEEKS
PLUS RACE-WEEK COUNTDOWN

 4-hour marathon is roughly 9:10 per mile. But **marathon-race pace** will be 9:00 per mile. (See "Marathon-Race Pace," page 60.)

Schedule for a 4:00 Marathon

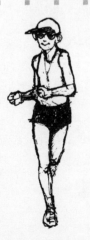

Weeks 1–8: Endurance Phase

WEEK 1:
    Monday—Jog 40 minutes.
    Tuesday—Cross train 30 minutes.
    Wednesday—Six x 400 meters at 2:05 to 2:15 pace.
    Thursday—Jog 30 minutes or rest.
    Friday—Cross train 20–30 minutes.
    Saturday—7 miles at 10:40 to 11:10 pace.
    Sunday—Rest.

WEEK 2:
>   Monday—Jog 40 minutes.
>   Tuesday—Cross train 30 minutes.
>   Wednesday—Eight x 400 meters at 2:05 to 2:15 pace.
>   Thursday—Jog 30 minutes or rest.
>   Friday—Cross train 30 minutes.
>   Saturday—9 miles at 10:40 to 11:10 pace.
>   Sunday—Rest.

WEEK 3:
>   Monday—Jog 40 minutes.
>   Tuesday—Cross train 30 minutes.
>   Wednesday—Ten x 400 meters at 2:05 to 2:15 pace.
>   Thursday—Jog 30 minutes or rest.
>   Friday—Cross train 30 minutes.
>   Saturday—11 miles at 10:40 to 11:20 pace.
>   Sunday—Rest.

WEEK 4:
>   Monday—Jog 40 minutes.
>   Tuesday—Cross train 30 minutes.
>   Wednesday—Twelve x 400 meters at 2:05 to 2:15 pace.
>   Thursday—Jog 40 minutes or rest.
>   Friday—Cross train 30 minutes.
>   Saturday—13 miles at 10:40 to 11:20 pace.
>   Sunday—Rest.

WEEK 5:
>   Monday—Jog 40 minutes.
>   Tuesday—Cross train 30 minutes.
>   Wednesday—Six x 400 meters at 2:00 to 2:10 pace.
>   Thursday—Jog 30 minutes or rest.
>   Friday—Cycle or swim 30 minutes.
>   Saturday—8 miles at 10:40 to 11:20 pace.
>   Sunday—Rest.

WEEK 6:

Monday—Jog 40 minutes.

Tuesday—Cross train 30 minutes.

Wednesday—Fourteen x 400 meters at 2:00 to 2:10 pace.

Thursday—Jog 30 minutes.

Friday—Cross train 30 minutes or rest.

Saturday—15 miles at 10:40 to 11:10 pace.

Sunday—Rest.

WEEK 7:

Monday—Jog 40 minutes.

Tuesday—Cross train 30 minutes.

Wednesday—Sixteen x 400 meters at 2:00 to 2:10 pace.

Thursday—Jog 30 minutes.

Friday—Cross train 30 minutes or rest.

Saturday—17 miles at 10:40 to 11:10 pace.

Sunday—Rest.

WEEK 8:

Monday—Jog 40 minutes.

Tuesday—Cross train 30 minutes.

Wednesday—Sixteen x 400 meters at 2:00 to 2:10 pace.

Thursday—Jog 30 minutes or rest.

Friday—Cross train 30 minutes.

Saturday—10 miles at 10:40 to 11:10 pace.

Sunday—Rest.

Weeks 9–14: Stamina Phase

WEEK 9:

Monday—Jog 40 minutes.

Tuesday—Cross train 30 minutes.

Wednesday—4 miles at 8:45 to 8:50 pace.

Thursday—Jog 30 minutes or rest.

Friday—Cross train 30 minutes.
Saturday—19 miles at 10:40 to 11:10 pace.
Sunday—Rest.

WEEK 10:
Monday—Jog 40 minutes.
Tuesday—Cross train 30 minutes.
Wednesday—6 miles at 8:45 to 8:50 pace.
Thursday—Jog 30 minutes or rest.
Friday—Rest.
Saturday—10 miles at 10:40 to 11:10 pace.
Sunday—Rest.

WEEK 11:
Monday—Rest.
Tuesday—Jog 30 minutes.
Wednesday—3 miles at 8:45 pace.
Thursday—Jog 30 minutes or rest.
Friday—Cross train 30 minutes.
Saturday—21 miles at 10:40 to 11:10 pace.
Sunday—Rest.

WEEK 12:
Monday—Jog 40 minutes.
Tuesday—Cross train 30 minutes.
Wednesday—7 miles at 8:45 to 8:50 pace.
Thursday—Jog 30 minutes or rest.
Friday—Rest.
Saturday—10 miles at 10:40 to 11:10 pace.
Sunday—Rest.

WEEK 13:
Monday—Rest.
Tuesday—Cross train 30 minutes.
Wednesday—8 miles at 8:45 to 8:50 pace.
Thursday—Jog 30 minutes or rest.

Friday—Rest.
Saturday—14 miles at 10:40 to 11:10 pace.
Sunday—Rest.

WEEK 14:
Monday—Jog 40 minutes.
Tuesday—Cross train 30 minutes.
Wednesday—8 miles at 8:45 to 8:50 pace.
Thursday—Jog 30 minutes.
Friday—Rest.
Saturday—3 miles at 10:40 to 11:10 pace.
Sunday—Rest.

Weeks 15 and 16: Taper Phase

WEEK 15:
Monday—Rest.
Tuesday—Cross train 30 minutes.
Wednesday—Jog 30 minutes.
Thursday—Cross train 30 minutes.
Friday—Jog 30 minutes.
Saturday—10 miles at 10:40 to 11:10 pace.
Sunday—Rest.

WEEK 16:
Monday: Jog 40 minutes.
Tuesday—Cross train 30 minutes.
Wednesday—5 miles at 9:00 pace—Marathon Pace!
Thursday—Jog 30 minutes.
Friday—Cross train 30 minutes.
Saturday—8 miles at 9:00 pace—Marathon Pace!
Sunday—Rest.

WEEK 17: MARATHON WEEK
Monday—Rest.
Tuesday—Jog 30 minutes.
Wednesday—4 miles at 9:00 pace—Marathon Pace!
Thursday—Rest.
Friday—Jog 20 minutes or rest.
Saturday—Rest.
Sunday—4-hour marathon!

------------------------------ MARATHON-RACE PACE ------------------------------

As you've noticed, marathon pace is slightly faster—about 10 seconds per mile faster—than the **exact pace** you need to run 26.2 miles to finish a marathon in **4 hours**.

This is because when you're running the marathon you want to build up a "cushion," that is, a time leeway, so you won't panic in the last 6 miles or so when you're slowing down a bit. (Almost everyone slows down.) If you have been running faster than exact pace, you can afford to run a bit slower toward the end of the race and not lose time.

Schedule for a 4:15 Marathon

Note: A 4:15 marathon is roughly 9:45 per mile. But **marathon race pace** will be 9:35 per mile.

Weeks 1-8: Endurance Phase

WEEK 1:
Monday—Jog 40 minutes.
Tuesday—Cross train 30 minutes.
Wednesday—Six x 400 meters at 2:10 to 2:20 pace.
Thursday—Cross train 30 minutes or rest.
Friday—Jog 20 minutes.
Saturday—7 miles at 10:45 to 11:15 pace.
Sunday—Rest.

WEEK 2:
Monday—Jog 40 minutes.
Tuesday—Cross train 30 minutes.
Wednesday—Eight x 400 meters at 2:10 to 2:20 pace.
Thursday—Cross train 30 minutes or rest.
Friday—Jog 20 minutes.
Saturday—9 miles at 10:45 to 11:15 pace.
Sunday—Rest.

WEEK 3:
Monday—Jog 40 minutes.
Tuesday—Cross train 30 minutes.
Wednesday—Ten x 400 meters at 2:10 to 2:20 pace.
Thursday—Cross train 30 minutes or rest.
Friday—Jog 20 minutes.
Saturday—11 miles at 10:45 to 11:15 pace.
Sunday—Rest.

WEEK 4:
Monday—Jog 40 minutes.
Tuesday—Cross train 30 minutes.
Wednesday—Twelve x 400 meters at 2:10 to 2:20 pace.
Thursday—Cross train 30 minutes or rest.

Friday—Jog 20 minutes.
Saturday—13 miles at 10:45 to 11:15 pace.
Sunday—Rest.

WEEK 5:

Monday—Jog 40 minutes.
Tuesday—Cross train 30 minutes.
Wednesday—Six x 400 meters at 2:10 to 2:15 pace.
Thursday—Cross train 30 minutes or rest.
Friday—Jog 20 minutes.
Saturday—8 miles at 10:45 to 11:15 pace.
Sunday—Rest.

WEEK 6:

Monday—Jog 40 minutes.
Tuesday—Cross train 30 minutes.
Wednesday—Fourteen x 400 meters at 2:10 to 2:15 pace.
Thursday—Cross train 30 minutes or rest.
Friday—Jog 20 minutes.
Saturday—15 miles at 10:45 to 11:15 pace.
Sunday—Rest.

WEEK 7:

Monday—Jog 40 minutes.
Tuesday—Cross train 30 minutes.
Wednesday—Sixteen x 400 meters at 2:10 pace.
Thursday—Cross train 30 minutes or rest.
Friday—Jog 20 minutes.
Saturday—10 miles at 10:45 to 11:15 pace.
Sunday—Rest.

WEEK 8:

Monday—Jog 40 minutes.
Tuesday—Cross train 30 minutes.
Wednesday—Sixteen x 400 meters at 2:10 pace.
Thursday—Cross train 30 minutes or rest.

Friday—Jog 20 minutes.
Saturday—10 miles at 10:45 to 11:15 pace.
Sunday—Rest.

Weeks 9–14: Stamina Phase

WEEK 9:
Monday—Jog 40 minutes.
Tuesday—Cross train 30 minutes.
Wednesday—4 miles at 9:20 to 9:25 pace.
Thursday—Cross train 30 minutes or rest.
Friday—Jog 20 minutes.
Saturday—7 miles at 10:45 to 11:15 pace.
Sunday—Rest.

WEEK 10:
Monday—Jog 40 minutes.
Tuesday—Cross train 30 minutes.
Wednesday—5 miles at 9:20 to 9:25 pace.
Thursday—Cross train 30 minutes or rest.
Friday—Jog 20 minutes.
Saturday—10 miles at 10:45 to 11:15 pace.
Sunday—Rest.

WEEK 11:
Monday—Rest.
Tuesday—Cross train 30 minutes.
Wednesday—3 miles at 9:20 to 9:25 pace.
Thursday—Rest.
Friday—Jog 20 minutes.
Saturday—20 miles at 10:45 to 11:15 pace.
Sunday—Rest.

WEEK 12:
    Monday—Jog 40 minutes.
    Tuesday—Cross train 30 minutes.
    Wednesday—6 miles at 9:20 to 9:25 pace.
    Thursday—Cross train 30 minutes.
    Friday—Rest.
    Saturday—23 miles at 10:45 to 11:15 pace.
    Sunday—Rest.

WEEK 13:
    Monday—Rest.
    Tuesday—Jog 30 minutes.
    Wednesday—8 miles at 9:20 to 9:25 pace.
    Thursday—Cross train 30 minutes.
    Friday—Rest.
    Saturday—14 miles at 10:45 to 11:15 pace.
    Sunday—Rest.

WEEK 14:
    Monday—Jog 40 minutes.
    Tuesday—Cross train 30 minutes.
    Wednesday—8 miles at 9:20 to 9:25 pace.
    Thursday—Cross train 30 minutes or rest.
    Friday—Rest.
    Saturday—24 miles at 10:45 to 11:15 pace.
    Sunday—Rest.

Weeks 15 and 16: Taper Phase

WEEK 15:
    Monday—Rest.
    Tuesday—Cross train 30 minutes.
    Wednesday—Jog 30 minutes.
    Thursday—Cross train 30 minutes or rest.
    Friday—Jog 30 minutes.

Saturday—10 miles at 10:45 to 11:15 pace.
Sunday—Rest.

WEEK 16:
    Monday—Jog 40 minutes.
    Tuesday—Cross train 30 minutes.
    Wednesday—5 miles at 9:35 pace—Marathon Pace!
    Thursday—Rest.
    Friday—Cross train 30 minutes.
    Saturday—8 miles at 9:35 pace—Marathon Pace!
    Sunday—Rest.

WEEK 17: MARATHON WEEK!
    Monday—Rest.
    Tuesday—Jog 30 minutes.
    Wednesday—4 miles at 9:35 pace—Marathon Pace!
    Thursday—Rest.
    Friday—Jog 20 minutes or rest.
    Saturday—Rest.
    Sunday—4:15 marathon!

Schedule for a 4:30 Marathon

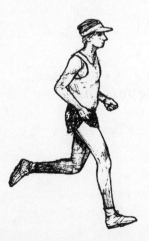

A 4:30 marathon is roughly 10:20 per mile. But marathon-race pace will be 10:10 per mile.

Weeks 1–8: Endurance Phase

WEEK 1:
    Monday—Jog 40 minutes.
    Tuesday—Cross train 30 minutes.

Wednesday—Six x 400 meters at 2:15 to 2:25.
Thursday—Cross train 30 minutes or rest.
Friday—Jog 30 minutes.
Saturday—7 miles at 11:50 to 12:20 pace.
Sunday—Rest.

WEEK 2:
Monday—Jog 40 minutes.
Tuesday—Cross train 30 minutes.
Wednesday—Seven x 400 meters at 2:15 to 2:25.
Thursday—Cross train 30 minutes or rest.
Friday—Jog 30 minutes.
Saturday—9 miles at 11:50 to 12:20 pace.
Sunday—Rest.

WEEK 3:
Monday—Jog 40 minutes.
Tuesday—Cross train 30 minutes.
Wednesday—Eight x 400 meters at 2:15 to 2:25 pace.
Thursday—Cross train 30 minutes or rest.
Friday—Jog 30 minutes.
Saturday—11 miles at 11:50 to 12:20 pace.
Sunday—Rest.

WEEK 4:
Monday—Jog 40 minutes.
Tuesday—Cross train 30 minutes.
Wednesday—Ten x 400 meters at 2:15 to 2:25 pace.
Thursday—Cross train 30 minutes or rest.
Friday—Jog 30 minutes.
Saturday—13 miles at 11:50 to 12:20 pace.
Sunday—Rest.

WEEK 5:
  Monday—Jog 40 minutes.
  Tuesday—Cross train 30 minutes.
  Wednesday—Six x 400 meters at 2:15 to 2:25 pace.
  Thursday—Cross train 30 minutes.
  Friday—Jog 30 minutes.
  Saturday—8 miles at 11:50 to 12:20 pace.
  Sunday—Rest.

WEEK 6:
  Monday—Jog 40 minutes.
  Tuesday—Cross train 30 minutes.
  Wednesday—Twelve x 400 meters at 2:15 to 2:25 pace.
  Thursday—Cross train 30 minutes or rest.
  Friday—Jog 30 minutes.
  Saturday—15 miles at 11:50 to 12:20 pace.
  Sunday—Rest.

WEEK 7:
  Monday—Jog 40 minutes.
  Tuesday—Cross train 30 minutes.
  Wednesday—Fourteen x 400 meters at 2:15 to 2:20 pace.
  Thursday—Cross train 30 minutes or rest.
  Friday—Jog 30 minutes.
  Saturday—17 miles at 11:50 to 12:20 pace.
  Sunday—Rest.

WEEK 8:
  Monday—Jog 40 minutes.
  Tuesday—Cross train 30 minutes.
  Wednesday—Sixteen x 400 meters at 2:15 pace.
  Thursday—Cross train 30 minutes or rest.
  Friday—Jog 30 minutes.
  Saturday—10 miles at 11:50 to 12:20 pace.
  Sunday—Rest.

Weeks 9–14: Stamina Phase

WEEK 9:

Monday—Jog 40 minutes.
Tuesday—Cross train 30 minutes.
Wednesday—5 miles at 9:55 to 10:00 pace.
Thursday—Cross train 30 minutes or rest.
Friday—Jog 30 minutes.
Saturday—19 miles at 11:50 to 12:20 pace.
Sunday—Rest.

WEEK 10:

Monday—Jog 40 minutes.
Tuesday—Cross train 30 minutes.
Wednesday—6 miles at 9:55 to 10:00 pace.
Thursday—Cross train 30 minutes or rest.
Friday—Jog 30 minutes.
Saturday—21 miles at 11:50 to 12:20 pace.
Sunday—Rest.

WEEK 11:

Monday—Rest.
Tuesday—Cross train 30 minutes.
Wednesday—3 miles at 9:55 to 10:00 pace.
Thursday—Cross train 30 minutes or rest.
Friday—Rest.
Saturday—10 miles at 11:50 to 12:20 pace.
Sunday—Rest.

WEEK 12:

Monday—Jog 40 minutes.
Tuesday—Cross train 30 minutes.
Wednesday—7 miles at 9:55 to 10:00 pace.
Thursday—Cross train 30 minutes or rest.
Friday—Rest.

Saturday—23 miles at 11:50 to 12:20 pace.
Sunday—Rest.

WEEK 13:

Monday—Jog 40 minutes.
Tuesday—Cross train 30 minutes.
Wednesday—8 miles at 9:55 to 10:00 pace.
Thursday—Cross train 30 minutes or rest.
Friday—Rest.
Saturday—14 miles at 11:50 to 12:20 pace.
Sunday—Rest.

WEEK 14:

Monday—Jog 40 minutes.
Tuesday—Cross train 30 minutes.
Wednesday—8 miles at 9:55 to 10:00 pace.
Thursday—Cross train 30 minutes or rest.
Friday—Rest.
Saturday—24 miles at 11:50 to 12:20 pace.
Sunday—Rest.

Weeks 15 and 16: Taper Phase

WEEK 15:

Monday—Rest.
Tuesday—Cross train 30 minutes.
Wednesday—Jog 30 minutes.
Thursday—Rest.
Friday—Jog 30 minutes.
Saturday—10 miles at 11:20 to 11:50 pace.
Sunday—Rest.

WEEK 16:

Monday—Jog 40 minutes.
Tuesday—Cross train 30 minutes.

Wednesday—5 miles at 10:10 pace—Marathon Pace!
Thursday—Rest.
Friday—Jog 30 minutes.
Saturday—8 miles at 10:10 pace—Marathon Pace!
Sunday—Rest.

WEEK 17: MARATHON WEEK
Monday—Rest.
Tuesday—Cross train 30 minutes.
Wednesday—5 miles at 10:10 pace—Marathon Pace!
Thursday—Rest.
Friday—Jog 20 minutes or rest.
Saturday—Rest.
Sunday—4:30 marathon!

Schedule for a 4:45 Marathon

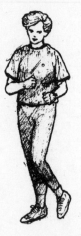

A 4:45 marathon is roughly 10:52 per mile. But marathon-race pace will be 10:42 per mile.

Weeks 1–8: Endurance Phase

WEEK 1:
Monday—Jog 40 minutes.
Tuesday—Cross train 30 minutes.
Wednesday—Six x 400 meters at 2:25 to 2:35 pace.
Thursday—Cross train 30 minutes or rest.
Friday—Jog 30 minutes.
Saturday—7 miles at 12:22 to 12:52 per mile pace.
Sunday—Rest.

WEEK 2:

    Monday—Jog 40 minutes.
    Tuesday—Cross train 30 minutes.
    Wednesday—Seven x 400 meters at 2:25 to 2:35 pace.
    Thursday—Cross train 30 minutes or rest.
    Friday—Jog 30 minutes.
    Saturday—9 miles at 12:22 to 12:52 pace.
    Sunday—Rest.

WEEK 3:

    Monday—Jog 40 minutes.
    Tuesday—Cross train 30 minutes.
    Wednesday—Eight x 400 meters at 2:25 to 2:35 pace.
    Thursday—Cross train 30 minutes or rest.
    Friday—Jog 30 minutes.
    Saturday—11 miles at 12:22 to 12:52 pace.
    Sunday—Rest.

WEEK 4:

    Monday—Jog 40 minutes.
    Tuesday—Cross train 30 minutes.
    Wednesday—Ten x 400 meters at 2:25 to 2:35 pace.
    Thursday—Cross train 30 minutes or rest.
    Friday—Jog 30 minutes.
    Saturday—13 miles at 12:22 to 12:52 pace.
    Sunday—Rest.

WEEK 5:

    Monday—Jog 40 minutes.
    Tuesday—Cross train 30 minutes.
    Wednesday—Six x 400 meters at 2:25 to 2:35 pace.
    Thursday—Cross train 30 minutes or rest.
    Friday—Jog 30 minutes.
    Saturday—8 miles at 12:22 to 12:52 pace.
    Sunday—Rest.

WEEK 6:

    Monday—Jog 40 minutes.
    Tuesday—Cross train 30 minutes.
    Wednesday—Twelve x 400 meters at 2:25 to 2:35 pace.
    Thursday—Cross train 30 minutes or rest.
    Friday—Jog 30 minutes.
    Saturday—15 miles at 12:22 to 12:52 pace.
    Sunday—Rest.

WEEK 7:

    Monday—Jog 40 minutes.
    Tuesday—Cross train 30 minutes.
    Wednesday—Fourteen x 400 meters at 2:25 to 2:30 pace.
    Thursday—Cross train 30 minutes or rest.
    Friday—Jog 30 minutes.
    Saturday—17 miles at 12:22 to 12:52 pace.
    Sunday—Rest.

WEEK 8:

    Monday—Jog 40 minutes.
    Tuesday—Cross train 30 minutes.
    Wednesday—Sixteen x 400 meters at 2:25 pace.
    Thursday—Rest.
    Friday—Jog 30 minutes.
    Saturday—10 miles at 12:22 to 12:52 pace.
    Sunday—Rest.

Weeks 9–14: Stamina Phase

WEEK 9:

    Monday—Jog 40 minutes.
    Tuesday—Cross train 30 minutes.
    Wednesday—5 miles at 10:25 to 10:30 pace.
    Thursday—Cross train 30 minutes or rest.
    Friday—Jog 30 minutes.

Saturday—19 miles at 12:22 to 12:52 pace.
Sunday—Rest.

WEEK 10:
 Monday—Jog 40 minutes.
 Tuesday—Cross train 30 minutes.
 Wednesday—6 miles at 10:25 to 10:30 pace.
 Thursday—Cross train 30 minutes or rest.
 Friday—Jog 30 minutes.
 Saturday—21 miles at 12:22 to 12:52 pace.
 Sunday—Rest.

WEEK 11:
 Monday—Rest.
 Tuesday—Cross train 30 minutes.
 Wednesday—3 miles at 10:25 to 10:30 pace.
 Thursday—Cross train 30 minutes or rest.
 Friday—Rest.
 Saturday—10 miles at 12:22 to 12:52 pace.
 Sunday—Rest.

WEEK 12:
 Monday—Jog 40 minutes.
 Tuesday—Cross train 30 minutes.
 Wednesday—7 miles at 10:25 to 10:30 pace.
 Thursday—Cross train 30 minutes or rest.
 Friday—Rest.
 Saturday—23 miles at 12:22 to 12:52 pace.
 Sunday—Rest.

WEEK 13:
 Monday—Jog 40 minutes.
 Tuesday—Cross train 30 minutes.
 Wednesday—8 miles at 10:25 to 10:30 pace.
 Thursday—Cross train 30 minutes or rest.
 Friday—Rest.

Saturday—14 miles at 12:22 to 12:52 pace.
Sunday—Rest.

WEEK 14:
Monday—Jog 40 minutes.
Tuesday—Cross train 30 minutes.
Wednesday—8 miles at 10:25 to 10:30 pace.
Thursday—Cross train 30 minutes or rest.
Friday—Rest.
Saturday—24 miles at 12:22 to 12:52 pace.
Sunday—Rest.

Weeks 15 and 16: Taper Phase

WEEK 15:
Monday—Rest.
Tuesday—Cross train 30 minutes.
Wednesday—Jog 30 minutes.
Thursday—Rest.
Friday—Jog 30 minutes.
Saturday—10 miles at 12:22 to 12:52 pace.
Sunday—Rest.

WEEK 16:
Monday—Jog 40 minutes.
Tuesday—Cross train 30 minutes.
Wednesday—5 miles at 10:42 pace—Marathon Pace!
Thursday—Rest.
Friday—Jog 30 minutes.
Saturday—8 miles at 10:42 pace—Marathon Pace!
Sunday—Rest.

WEEK 17: MARATHON WEEK
Monday—Rest.
Tuesday—Cross train 30 minutes.

Wednesday—5 miles at 10:42 pace—Marathon Pace!
Thursday—Rest.
Friday—Jog 20 minutes or rest.
Saturday—Rest.
Sunday— 4:45 marathon!

Day-by-day marathon training is the meat and potatoes of your marathon preparation. Now let's turn to how to handle the **4-hour marathon** itself.

eight

MISSION POSSIBLE

Your mission, Mr. Pheidippedes . . .
Now we come to the race itself—the trek made famous when the Greek messenger Pheidippedes ran from the battlefield of Marathon to Athens with news of victory.

Mile-by-Mile Marathon Checklist

START: Go slow, with your arms out to guard against being bumped and knocked off balance. Don't weave in and out of other runners. It will only waste energy or you'll end up on the pavement. Relax. This is your warm-up.

HALF-MILE TO ONE MILE: The field starts to clear out. Find 9:00 pace. Move to an open lane. Soak in the atmosphere of the race and store it for the end. Tell yourself:

I'm running a marathon in **4 hours!** I'm running a marathon in **4 hours!**

ONE MILE: You should be at a 9:10 to 9:15 pace. Your time might be a little slower—maybe 10 to 20 seconds slower—because of the crowd at the start. Don't panic. You will make up time. Stay relaxed. Cruise.

MILE TWO: Elapsed time: 18:05–18:10. Most of the runners around you will be 4-hour runners. A few will not be. They will be speeding by to catch their friends who are after 3:30 marathons. Or they might be lost souls who you will pass somewhere between 10 and 20 miles as they struggle for breath. Let them go. Stick to your pace. You know what you have to do. Stick to it.

MILE THREE: 27:00. FIRST WATER STOP. Drink. (See "Boys & Girls," below.)

-------------------------------- BOYS & GIRLS --------------------------------

   Water stops at marathons are a world unto themselves, little oases that can seem like mirages toward the end of a marathon. At most marathons they come every 2 to 3 miles. (And some marathons have them every mile after 20 miles: Call ahead and find out where the water stops will be so you can simulate them in your long training runs.) Each of these water stops is like jogging through a cafeteria line where one or two things are offered—just water or water and an energy drink. Water stops have a protocol that you need to follow if you want to make sure you don't come away thirsty:

1. Spot the water stop early: There could be signs reading "Water Stop Ahead" or someone yelling to you that one is ahead.

2. Make your choice: Water usually comes first at a stop that offers both water and an energy drink. You should take water early, and energy drinks and water later (after six miles, about forty-five minutes into your marathon).

3. Slow down.

4. Line up. Make a single- or double-file line as you head into the water stop. Get close to the side where they're handing out water.

5. Go for a drink early. Major water stops can be as long as 30 yards. If you're running in a group, go for water early in the stop. That way if—heaven forbid!—you should drop your cup, you can always get another shot later down the line. (Note: If you miss your water entirely, you should stop and go back. Don't skip a water stop, ever—even the early ones, when you're not thirsty yet. These, in fact, are most important because the water you take early will help you later.)

6. Make eye contact early: Pick a volunteer who is holding out a water cup and make eye contact with him or her. Hold out your hand to signal that you want water.

7. Grab the cup and then center it in front of you. Some will spill out. Get your balance. Move away from the congested water stop area. Slow down—or stop if necessary. Crush the cup so you make a funnel. And drink it down.

8. On hot days you may want to grab another cup to pour over your head, but just make sure it's water and don't pour so much on you that you soak your shoes.

9. Throw the cup in the barrels down the road or pitch it to the side.

10. Get back into your 9:00 pace. Don't sprint to make up for lost time—it's only a few seconds. You will make that up in the next mile.

What you want to consume at each water station is this:

Before 45 minutes into the marathon: Drink water.

After 45 minutes: Alternate water and energy drink every other stop.

If you're taking **fuel** (an energy gel, glucose tablet, candy, cookie or energy bar), take them at every other water station after one hour . . . with plenty of water.

MILE FOUR: You should be close to 36:00, our designated marathon pace. Concentrate on relaxing. These next miles should pass by quickly.

MILE FIVE: 45:00. Great! Right on pace. Shake out your arms a little. Turn your head from side to side. Stay loose and smooth.

MILE SIX: 54:00. Prepare for the next water station. Take water or an energy drink. **Fuel.**

MILE SEVEN: One hour and three minutes. **First crisis point!** You've completed a 10K. You've gotten a lift from an energy drink or gel or bar. You're cruising along at marathon pace. It feels so good. So easy. You see runners up the road and a little voice inside your head says: "Go for it. Pick up the pace!"

No. No. No. Treat the urge to pick up the pace during a marathon like Noel Coward treated the urge to exercise: "I sat down until the feeling passed."

You've trained to run at a 9:00 pace. Speeding up might feel good for a while but you're only setting yourself up for a drastic slowdown later in the race.

Hold the pace!

MILE EIGHT: 1:12:00. Good. You've resisted the urge to speed up. Get back into the groove. Your race is more than one-fourth over and you are still very fresh. Relax.

MILE NINE: 1:21:00. Stay in the groove and prepare for the next water stop. Take water this time. Make sure you drink plenty.

MILE TEN: 1:30:00. Ten miles into the race. Remember back three months ago when 10 miles was your long run?! Dwell on your newfound endurance. Relax.

MILE ELEVEN: 1:39:00. Do a body check. Start by concentrating on your feet, then legs, back, arms and head. All still there? All still intact? Of course. Then carry on. Relax.

RACE-DAY ATTIRE: THE THREE LEVELS OF DRESS

Moderate to warm weather—high 50s to 70s—marathons are pretty easy to dress for: shorts and a singlet.

But when the thermometer drops below the mid-50s you need to think about dressing for the three parts of the marathon.

1. The first is the start, where you will be standing for half an hour or so before you even start moving. If it's cold, you'll need a "throwaway" shirt to cover yourself with at the start and during the early miles. You just take it off when you heat up and pitch it to the side of the road. (Some runners even use plastic garbage bags. They cut out arm holes and put the bags on like Halloween costumes. They may look funny, but they serve the purpose.)

2. The second part is the majority of the race itself, say, from 3 miles to 20 miles. This is when you're grooving. Running well. You want to be comfortable, with no excess clothes. You see yourself as an elite runner who only needs a singlet and shorts, and the temptation will be to dress as such, even when it's cooler than 50 degrees. But don't—because you also have to take into account the final part of the marathon . . .

3. The last 6 miles. If the temperature is below 50 degrees, the last hour of your marathon will feel much colder than the first three hours. That's a natural reaction to the fatigue, stress and dehydration of running that long. So don't strip down to a singlet and shorts if it's cold and you feel good at, say, mile 5. Remember you have a long way to go.

MILE 12: 1:48:00. Almost halfway. Take an energy drink or **fuel** and water. Relax.

MILE 13: 1:57:00. Check pace and look ahead for the half-marathon marker. Relax.

HALF-MARATHON: 1:58:00. Great! On pace—with a two-minute cushion.

MILE 14: 2:06:00. **Second crisis point!** The half-marathon felt so good and smooth. That little voice is saying again: Why not pick up the pace? You can run a 3:55 or faster. Go for it!
No. No. No. Keep holding back. Stay the course.

MILE 15: 2:15:00. Good. You beat temptation. Time for water. **Fuel.** Back on pace. Relax. Stay focused.

MILE 16: 2:24:00. Ten miles to go!

MILE 17: 2:33:00. Stay relaxed. Focused. Shake out your arms.

MILE 18: 2:42:00. Next water station: Energy drink or **fuel** and water.

48 HOURS

Your marathon training started 4 months ago, but a crucial time that goes with the race itself is the final 48 hours before the marathon. Here's your countdown for things you should keep in mind:

48–36 hours: Do your traveling now.

36–24 hours: Sleep in two days before. The night before a marathon will be a fitful night of sleep because of nerves and anticipation, so make sure that two nights before you get a good eight to nine hours sleep. If you can, take a nap that afternoon, too.

24–12 hours: Stay off your feet. Don't cruise the marathon expo for hours or go shopping with friends. Find a spot and plant it. At home or in your hotel room, with your feet up. Keep your fluid level up by drinking water every half hour or so—especially if you flew in to the race, because flying can dehydrate your body. (It's also a good idea to take a water bottle with you on the flight.)

12 hours: Lay out your race stuff the night before. Shoes, socks, singlet with race number, gloves (if needed), hat, etc. You don't want to waste energy rushing around to find your race singlet when you've got a marathon to run in an hour! (See "Race-Day Attire," pp. 81–82.)

10 hours: Early to bed, early to rise. Get to bed early even if you don't feel like sleeping. Bring a book. Watch a movie. Don't hang out and burn nervous energy.

3 hours: The morning of the race, try the two-hour rule. Get up at least two hours before the race, three hours if you have to drive 45 minutes to get there. (A good rule of thumb: If you have to drive more than 45 minutes the morning of the marathon, get there one or two days before.) The first thing on your mind should be fuel. Eat your favorite pre–long run meal that you came up with during training.

1 hour to 45 minutes: Arrive at the starting area. Go to the bathroom now. Drink a few more ounces but don't fill your stomach so much that the bathroom suddenly seems more important than the starting line.

30 minutes: Locate your starting spot. Stretch. Resist the urge to jog for 20 minutes. You'll warm up in the first few miles of the marathon.

15 minutes: Get to your starting spot. Shake out your arms. Check energy tablets, gel or candies, if you're using them. Recheck shoelaces. Shake hands with training partners.

10 minutes: Repeat race plan in your head. Go over your splits. Give yourself a boost of confidence.

5 minutes: Think about the last four months of training. You are ready to run a **4-hour marathon!**

1 minute: Put your watch in stopwatch mode. Get ready to run.

MILE 19: 2:51:00. Stay focused. Concentrate now. Eight miles to go!

MILE 20: 3:00:00. A 10K to go! And you've got more than a minute and a half in the bank. Fatigue might be setting in. But remind yourself that you went farther than this on your Saturday morning long runs several times. You are going to run a **4-hour marathon!**

MILE 21: 3:09:00. Water and fuel. **Final crisis point!** You have broken through "the Wall" and don't feel that bad. Time to pick up the pace, right?
  No. No. No. Keep the pace. Keep the pace.

MILE 22: 3:18:00. Look for more water and **fuel**. Four miles to go!

MILE 23: 3:27:00. Look for more water and **fuel**. Maintain! Maintain! Think back to the 4 months of marathon training. The days when you ran in the rain or snow. The days when you got out of bed at dawn. You can do it. You can do it.
  Slow down a bit if you have to, but resist that urge to stop. Once you do, it will be harder to get going again. Remember: You've built up a cushion of time so you can relax the pace and still come in under **4 hours.**

KRAMER VERSUS KRAMER:
THE *SEINFELD* COUNTDOWN

There are many ways of mentally getting through the last miles of a marathon. Run with friends, sing a song, enjoy the scenery or work out a math problem in your head. One way for **4-hour marathoners** to finish the last half hour is what's called the *Seinfeld* Countdown.

In other words, think of the last 30 minutes of your marathon as an episode of *Seinfeld*.

30 minutes to go: Right now we've got the teaser. Or if it's an old show, Jerry is doing his monologue. Remember the one about . . .

25 minutes to go: Kramer stumbles in the door now, skidding on the floor. He's got a get-rich-quick scheme. What is it? You make it up.

20 minutes: Elaine is worried about . . . (fill in the blank). Example: the color of her socks.

15 minutes: Jerry can't get . . . (fill in the blank). Example: toast the way he wants it.

10 minutes: George is upset because . . . (fill in the blank). Example: he has too much nose hair.

5 minutes: Boy, if only these people would run a marathon, right?

1 minute: Now we're ready for all the plots to come together. Kind of like the end of training **4 months** for a **4-hour marathon**.

MILE 24: 3:36:00. Look for water. Concentrate. Lower your arms. Picture the finish line ahead. Imagine yourself in a hot shower and getting a cold drink.

MILE 25: 3:45:00. One mile to go. You are going to do it.

MILE 26: 3:54:00. Less than a quarter mile to go. Less than one lap around the track—remember all those 400-meter repeats you ran months ago? This last stretch will seem to take a long time. But instead of fighting it, drink it in. You are running a marathon in 4 hours! You are running a marathon in 4 hours!

26.2 MILES: 3:56:00. Spot the clock and revel in your accomplishment. You did it!

Mile Splits for 4:00, 4:15, 4:30 and 4:45 Marathons

Splits are something to go over in your head before the start of the race. Some runners write key splits for 1, 5, 10, 15, 20 and 25 miles on their arms in ink. Or even all their splits. The only problem with that is that once your arm gets sweaty, the ink can run. A hospital-type wristband is used by more and more runners to write down their mile splits and keep them handy. Believe me, it's hard to do the math in your head when you get past 20 miles. And if you have your splits written down, it's one less thing you have to concentrate on in those critical last miles.

Mile Splits for a 4:00 Marathon
(Race pace is 9:00)

Mile 1: 9:00	Mile 11: 1:39:00	Mile 20: 3:00:00
Mile 2: 18:00	Mile 12: 1:48:00	Mile 21: 3:09:00
Mile 3: 27:00	Mile 13: 1:57:00	Mile 22: 3:18:00
Mile 4: 36:00	Half-Marathon: 1:58:00	Mile 23: 3:27:00
Mile 5: 45:00	Mile 14: 2:06:00	Mile 24: 3:36:00
Mile 6: 54:00	Mile 15: 2:15:00	Mile 25: 3:45:00
Mile 7: 63:00	Mile 16: 2:24:00	Mile 26: 3:54:00
Mile 8: 72:00	Mile 17: 2:33:00	FINISH: 3:56:00
Mile 9: 81:00	Mile 18: 2:42:00	
Mile 10: 1:30:00	Mile 19: 2:51:00	

Mile Splits for a 4:15 Marathon
(Race pace is 9:35)

Mile 1: 9:35 to 9:45	Mile 9: 86:15	Mile 18: 2:52:30
Mile 2: 19:10 to 19:15	Mile 10: 95:50	Mile 19: 3:02:05
Mile 3: 28:45	Mile 11: 1:45:25	Mile 20: 3:11:40
Mile 4: 38:20	Mile 12: 1:55:00	Mile 21: 3:21:15
Mile 5: 47:55	Mile 13: 2:04:35	Mile 22: 3:30:50
Mile 6: 57:30	Half-Marathon: 2:05:32	Mile 23: 3:40:25
Mile 7: 67:05	Mile 14: 2:14:10	Mile 24: 3:50:00
Mile 8: 76:40	Mile 15: 2:23:45	Mile 25: 3:59:35
	Mile 16: 2:33:20	Mile 26: 4:09:10
	Mile 17: 2:42:55	FINISH: 4:11:05

Mile Splits for 4:30 Marathon
(Race pace is 10:10)

Mile 1: 10:10
Mile 2: 20:20
Mile 3: 30:30
Mile 4: 40:40
Mile 5: 50:50
Mile 6: 61:00
Mile 7: 71:10
Mile 8: 81:20
Mile 9: 1:31:30
Mile 10: 1:41:40

Mile 11: 1:51:50
Mile 12: 2:02:00
Mile 13: 2:12:10
Half-Marathon: 2:13:11
Mile 14: 2:22:20
Mile 15: 2:32:30
Mile 16: 2:42:40
Mile 17: 2:52:50
Mile 18: 3:03:00
Mile 19: 3:13:10

Mile 20: 3:23:30
Mile 21: 3:33:30
Mile 22: 3:43:40
Mile 23: 3:53:50
Mile 24: 4:04:00
Mile 25: 4:14:10
Mile 26: 4:24:20
FINISH: 4:26:22

Mile Splits for 4:45 Marathon
(Race pace is 10:42)

Mile 1: 10:42
Mile 2: 21:24
Mile 3: 32:06
Mile 4: 42:48
Mile 5: 53:30
Mile 6: 64:12
Mile 7: 74:54
Mile 8: 85:36
Mile 9: 96:18
Mile 10: 1:47:00

Mile 11: 1:57:42
Mile 12: 2:08:24
Mile 13: 2:19:06
Half-Marathon: 2:20:10
Mile 14: 2:29:48
Mile 15: 2:40:30
Mile 16: 2:51:12
Mile 17: 3:01:54
Mile 18: 3:12:36
Mile 19: 3:23:18

Mile 20: 3:34:00
Mile 21: 3:44:42
Mile 22: 3:55:24
Mile 23: 4:06:06
Mile 24: 4:16:48
Mile 25: 4:27:30
Mile 26: 4:38:12
FINISH: 4:40:20

Post-Marathon Countdown: 24 Hours

0–5 minutes: Walk through the finish chute. A volunteer will tear your tag—with your name—from your race number. Keep walking. Drink water or energy drinks. Find your friends and relatives.

10–45 minutes: Walk and wrap finish blanket around you if the weather is cool or not (you will cool down fast). Eat post-race carbs. Race organizers should have set up tables with bananas, cookies, etc. Just in case, you can ask friends or relatives to bring something for you to eat—and even sweats to wear until you get home or back to your hotel. If your stomach is upset, drink plenty of energy drinks instead of eating solid foods.

1–3 hours: Take a hot shower and enjoy a carbohydrate-rich meal with friends and training partners. Time to celebrate!

3–5 hours: Nap time.

5–12 hours: Travel if you have to. But if you've been smart, take this time to sightsee if you're in a new town.

12–20 hours: Sleep. Ahhh.

20–24 hours: Have breakfast. Read the newspaper articles about yesterday's marathon. Look for your name in the published race results.

The Week After

Treat the marathon like an extra-long run. That is, give yourself plenty of time to **recover** from it. A good rule of thumb is one day per mile raced, so you're looking at 26 days of recovery. During this time you should run no more than 8 miles at a time. And during this time you should be **refueling** your muscles with plenty of carbohydrates.

The first week is crucial. And it is outlined here.

Monday—Rest.
Tuesday—Cross train or rest.
Wednesday—Rest.
Thursday—Cross train 20 minutes or rest.
Friday—Rest.
Saturday—Jog 20 minutes or rest.
Sunday—Rest.

Again, the cardinal rule is to rest if you feel you need it. Don't force yourself back on your feet or you'll delay recovery.

In this chapter you've learned what to do before, during and after your **4-hour marathon**. But you still need to know more to make it to the finish line in 4 hours.

nine

SOCK DRAWER

Other Things You Need to Know to Run a 4-Hour Marathon

DO YOUR SATURDAY LONG RUNS "ON TIME": This means if the marathon you are targeting—and you need to target a marathon before you begin your training—begins at 8:00 A.M. in your same time zone, then you should do your long runs at 8:00 A.M. That means you should also practice your pre-race routine—getting up ahead of time to eat and drink. By working out this way your time clock and your body get in sync. Similarly, if your marathon starts two time zones west at 8:00 A.M. then your long runs should be done at 10:00 A.M. Get it? Good.

PACK LIGHT: Anxiety before your marathon is inevitable. So you want to do everything you can to keep any additional anxiety in check. One of the best ways—if you are flying to your marathon—is to pack everything in carry-on bags so you're assured that it will all get there. Or, if that can't be done, pack *all your essential running gear* in your carry-on bag. That way, you won't be worried about losing your shoes, shorts and singlet on the way to the race.

COLDS AND FLU: Generally any sort of sniffles, scratchy throat or cough is a sign that you should take a day or two off (it won't affect your fitness level). But if those symptoms also come with a fever and body aches, be *sure* to take three or four days off. You can—though it's not advised—run through a mild cold, that is, run with the cold until it is over. But many a runner who has tried to run through the onslaught of the flu has found himself or herself bedridden for a week. When in doubt, rest a few days and then jog easily. Besides, for runners the beginnings of a cold or flu is a sign that you're overdoing it. So why not heed the call?

Weight a Minute

You might want to supplement your marathon training with weight training, but make it light. That is, not more than two times a week. Two sets max (12 repetitions is a set) and with light weights (a weight you can lift another six or seven times after you're finished). Weight training will help strengthen your legs and whole body, and a stronger you can only help propel you to a **4-hour marathon**.

But beware of heavy weights, those that make you grunt and strain.

Training for a **4-hour marathon** is hard enough without lifting heavy weights. Besides, a hard weight workout becomes a hard workout and that cuts into your recovery days.

A good sample weight workout is a circuit, a lap around the weight room. The following descriptions of exercises are to be used with machines normally found in weight rooms. See a trainer if you have further questions.

The 4-Hour Marathoner's Weight Workout

These exercises are done on machines. If you have never used the machines at your gym before, ask for assistance from the staff so you can be sure you are using the equipment properly and are using the correct weight resistance.

1. Leg curl: Lie on your stomach with your knees just over the edge of the bench and your Achilles tendons hitting the roller pads. Hold the side grips to prevent your body from sliding. Curl your legs upward, trying to touch the roller pads to your butt. Pause. Lower slowly. If you feel any strain on your lower back, try one leg at a time. (Note: Hamstring strength is what you use for each stride.)

2. Leg extension: Place your ankles underneath the roller pads. Place hands on side grips for stability. Raise both legs until knees are straight (not locked at the knee). Pause. Lower slowly. (Note: Quadriceps strength helps balance out your leg strength and is the key to avoiding knee injuries.)

3. Calf raise: Put belt around your hips and stand up. Grab bar in front of you for stability. Raise up on both feet until you're on your toes. Pause. Lower slowly. (Note: Strong calf muscles are what you use to push off with each stride.)

4. Chest press: Lie flat on your back on the bench, feet flat on the floor and handles in line with your shoulders. With a wide grip, press up until your arms are extended. Pause.

Lower slowly. (Note: A strong chest helps carry the arms in the later stages of the marathon.)

5 Lat pulldown: Sit with thighs under roller pads for stability. Hold bar behind and slightly above your head with hands about shoulder-width apart. Lower bar behind your head to your shoulders. Pause. Raise slowly. (Note: A strong upper back helps keep the chest forward so you can breathe deeply.)

6 Lower back extension: Sit in the machine with thighs under the roller pads for stability and belt fastened around your waist. Place hands on upper thighs. Push torso backward slowly, as far as you can go. Pause. Return slowly. (Note: A strong lower back is the key to upright posture and efficient stride.)

7 Biceps curl: Sit in the machine with arms outstretched. Grab the handles and bring both arms back toward your shoulders. Pause. Lower slowly. (Note: Strong arms can help you pump your way to faster turnover workouts.)

8 Triceps curl: Sit in the machine with elbows higher than shoulders and arms bent back toward your head. Push on the roller pads with your closed hands to straighten your arms. Pause. Return slowly. (Note: Strong arms help balance your stride, especially in the later miles of the marathon.)

9 Crunches: Sit back in the machine with your hands grasping the handles. Take a deep breath, and exhale while you lean forward at the waist. Be sure to use your stomach muscles, not your arms, to pull the weight. Pause. Return slowly. (Note: Strong stomach muscles help guard against lower back strains in marathoners.)

10 Side bends: Sit upright in the machine with arms behind the roller pads and feet crossed in front of you. Looking

straight ahead, twist at the waist until you feel the muscles working. Pause. Return slowly. Repeat set, twisting to the other side. (Note: Strong side muscles will help keep your torso pointing forward when you run.)

As with heavy running workouts, weight lifting should be cut back or cut out in the last two to three weeks before your **4-hour marathon**. And cut out completely in the final week.

FRIENDS

Friends and family have come to the marathon to cheer you on. But where do they go? Everyone mills about the start, but unless it's a small marathon you won't be able to see them there. Good spots are the half-marathon or **anywhere in the last eight miles of the race.** This is when you'll need their support the most. So maybe they might want to position themselves at 20 miles to cheer you. Or, if they're running friends, they could **run in** with you until a half-mile from the finish, then drop off since they did not enter the marathon. This can be a great lift in the later stages of the marathon. And next year, when they run their **4-hour marathon,** you can return the favor.

Stretch It Out

The best time to stretch during training is *not* right before you run. It is better to wait until after you run, when the muscles are warm and loose, than to risk straining a muscle by stretching it when it's cold.

However, on your Wednesday turnover and tempo runs, you should warm up by jogging first. Then stretch before you start running fast. Also, it is best not to stretch right after a long run (anything over 12 miles) because the muscles will be tired and more susceptible to a strain.

With all stretches, you are *stretching,* not *pulling.* If you start to feel a strain, back off. The idea is to hold for 10 seconds (do not bounce), working up to 45 seconds. By stretching out your muscles you increase stride length (and therefore ease of running faster) and prevent against injuries.

The five basic marathoner's stretches are as follows:

1 Hamstring stretch: Keeping your right leg straight, place your left leg up on a chair or picnic table about halfway between knee and hip level. Lean toward your left foot with your *whole torso* (bending from the hip, not bending at the back) and hold. Repeat for the right leg.

2 Calf stretch: Stand about three feet from a wall. Stretch your right foot out behind you and keep your leg straight and foot on the floor. Have your left foot underneath you and your left knee bent. Place your palms on the wall and lean into the stretch. Hold. Repeat with the left leg.

3 Soleus stretch: Stand six inches from the wall. Put all your weight on your right foot and bend in toward the wall with your right knee, keeping your right foot flat. Hold. Repeat with the left leg. (Note: The soleus is the lower half of your calf and doesn't get stretched with the calf stretch.)

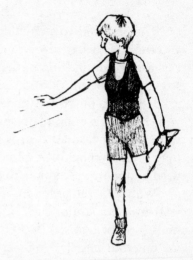

4 Quadriceps stretch: Stand on your right leg and bend your left leg backward at the knee. Grab your left ankle with your right hand and bring it up toward your left buttock. Hold. Keep back straight. Repeat for right leg. (Note: You might want to steady yourself by grabbing on to something with your left hand.)

5 Lower back and hip stretch: Lie on your back with your right knee bent and your left leg straight. Pull your right knee toward your chest. Hold. Repeat with the left leg. (Also, you can get a good back stretch by simply hanging from a pull-up bar. Grab the bar with both hands and lift your feet off the ground. Hold your back straight and feel the stretch.)

First Aid

Following is a concise guide to prevention, diagnosis and treatment for running injuries.

You can cut your chances of suffering a running injury in half if you follow these seven preventative procedures:

1. Don't run in worn-out shoes.

2. Run on soft surfaces.

3. Gradually build up the intensity and duration of your hard workouts.

4. Take your rest days seriously.

5. Cross train once or twice a week.

6. Strengthen your leg muscles with weight training.

7. Stretch several times a week.

Even by following preventive measures, you can still get injured. The key to dealing with any injury is to identify your injury and treat it right away.

In general, any twinge, twitch or tingle could be an indication that something is going wrong. The first step is to cancel that day's run and examine the injury more closely. If there is swelling, ice it for 20 minutes four times a day. (The best way to ice an injury is to use "ice cups"—frozen water in paper cups. Keeping the ice in the cup, rub the ice over the affected area. A bag of frozen peas is also an effective ice pack.) At this time you also should examine the injury more closely. Many times you will find that it has nothing to do with the injuries below, and by the time you've iced it for a third time the pain is gone—and it doesn't come back. (If you have an acute [sudden] twist or injury use the ICE method—ice, compression, elevation. If pain persists see your doctor.)

Yet that pain could be the beginning of a more serious injury, like the **five most common running injuries** listed below:

Iliotibial Band Syndrome

What Is It? Pain and inflammation on the outside of the knee. The IT band is a ligament that runs along the outside of the thigh. Pain and swelling happen when the band rubs against the femur bone at the knee.

How Do I Know If I've Got It? IT band syndrome is a dull ache that strikes a mile or two into your run. It will linger but disappear soon after your run. In severe cases, pain can be sharp and swelling can be so severe that your knee joint will be tender and swollen.

What Can I Do? Stop running. Apply ice four times a day for 20 minutes each time. Take aspirin or ibuprofen. Stretch the IT band: Stand with your right leg crossed in back of your left and extend your left arm against the wall. Lean toward the wall, while pushing your right hip out. Hold for 45 seconds. Repeat five times, three times a day.

Plantar Fascitis

What Is It? Pain and swelling on the bottom of the foot. The fascia—which has torn and is inflamed—is a fibrous band of tissue that runs from the heel to the toes.

How Do I Know If I've Got It? It feels like a bruise on your heel and is most severe in the morning when you get out of bed or at the beginning of a run. Your fascia is less flexible at those times. The pain, however, may fade once you start moving.

What Can I Do About It? Cut back on your running. Take aspirin or ibuprofen daily. Ice the area for 20 minutes four

times a day by rolling the arch of your foot over an un-
wrapped ice cup. Once the pain is gone, stretch your calf
muscles four times a day. Stretch the fascia by curling a towel
with your toes.

Chondromacacia

What Is It? A wearing away of the cartilage under the
kneecap, which causes pain and inflammation.

How Do I Know If I've Got It? Pain beneath or on the sides
of the kneecap. Most acute if you've run on a hilly road or
trail. In severe cases, you can feel grinding as rough cartilage
rubs against cartilage when knee is flexed.

What Can I Do About It? Stop running. Ice the knee four
times a day for 20 minutes. Take aspirin or ibuprofen. Once
the pain is gone, stretch and strengthen quadriceps.

Achilles Tendonitis

What Is It? Pain and swelling of the Achilles tendon from
small tears. The Achilles tendon is the strong tendon that con-
nects the calf muscles to the back of the heel bone.

How Do I Know If I've Got It? Dull or sharp pain along the
tendon. Can also involve redness or heat. And in severe cases
a cracking sound—not from the joint but along the tendon—
when the ankle moves.

What Can I Do About It? Stop running. Take aspirin or
ibuprofen daily. Ice the area four times a day for 20 minutes
each time. Once pain is gone, stretch the calf muscles.

Shin Splints

What Is It? Pain and swelling of tendons or muscles along the front of the shinbone.

How Do I Know If I've Got It? Dull pain at first, felt in the general area after a run. Eventually leads to tender spots on the front of the shin. If left untreated, can lead to stress fractures of the shinbone.

What Can I Do About It? Cut back on your running. Ice the area four times a day for 20 minutes each time. Take aspirin or ibuprofen. Stretch the calf muscles.

If self-treatment does not work in two weeks, see a sports doctor for other treatments. But, again, your best treatment is the preventative tips outlined above.

In this chapter you learned everything else you needed to know about running a **4-hour marathon**. But there is still one topic to cover: What marathon will you run?

ten

COURSE CONSCIOUS

This chapter is devoted to picking the marathon that you will run. As noted in chapter one, the course itself can be just as important to your training if you want to run a marathon in 4 hours.

First we'll look at some things to consider when choosing which marathon to run. Then we make the choice easier by listing dozens of fast courses.

Marathon Questions

Here are the four questions you need answered before you commit to a particular marathon.

1 Is it a fast course? There are dozens of fast marathon courses in the United States. Chicago, almost entirely flat, is one. The Cal International Marathon, which slopes slightly downhill, is another. Pick a marathon that is flat or slightly rolling or downhill.

2 What's the weather? Preferably temperatures between the 40s and the low 60s. Call the officials for the marathon you are considering. They keep records of average daily temperatures for marathon day.

3 How far away is it? Limit travel to three hours by car or plane (unless you can spend more than three days getting to and from the race). Any farther and you'll be "traveled out" before you get to the starting line. Also try to pick a marathon that's in your time zone or just one time zone away. That way you're not "off" your clock when the marathon starts.

4 How many runners? Two rules: No Godzillas. No foreign legion specials. Big marathons like New York City and Honolulu—both over 25,000 runners—are fun if you're an elite runner or want the experience of running them. But if you want to run a **4-hour marathon**, pick a mid-size marathon with a couple of hundred to several thousand runners. That way you're not running through a crowded bar-like atmosphere for most of the race, but you still have others around you to keep mentally in it. In that respect too, don't pick a flat marathon in Saskatchewan that has eight runners, or you'll find yourself at 21 miles, hungry, thirsty, tired—and all alone.

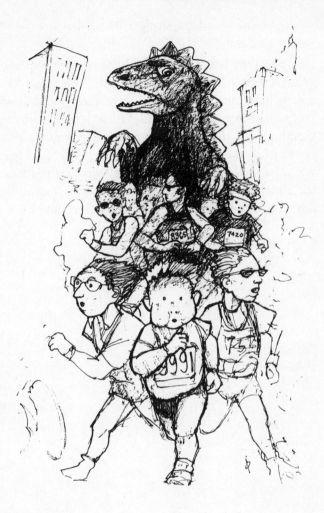

---------------------------- ERNIE'S TIP ----------------------------

"I ran my best marathon (3:45) on the fast course at Grandma's Marathon in Duluth," he says. "The course had a few rolls in it but was mostly flat. It was perfect weather, mid 50s, and we had a slight tailwind. Coming into town the last few miles, I got a good boost from the crowds there. Runners had told me it was a good course to run, and they were right. Picking the right marathon, like Grandma's was for me that day, can take minutes off your marathon time."

Recommended Marathons for
4-Hour Marathoners

All of these marathons would make a great venue for your 4-hour marathon. For a complete list of marathons in North America, and because dates and info are subject to change, consult marathonguide.com.

Then count back four months and start training!

There is no time requirement or previous racing experience for any of these marathons. The Boston Marathon in April is the only marathon where you have to qualify.

JANUARY
HP Houston Marathon
(Houston, Texas)
713-957-3453
hphoustonmarathon.com

ING Miami Marathon
(Miami, Florida)
305-278-8668
ingmiamimarathon.com

Rock'n'Roll Arizona
(Phoenix, Arizona)
858-450-6510
rnraz.com

Walt Disney World
    Marathon
(Orlando, Florida)
407-939-7810
disney.go.com

FEBRUARY
Cow Town Marathon
(Fort Worth, Texas)
817-735-2033
cowtownmarathon.org

Freescale Austin
    Marathon
(Austin, Texas)
512-478-4265
freescaleaustinmarathon
    .com

Mardi Gras Marathon
(New Orleans, Louisiana)
866-454-6561
mardigrasmarathon.com

MARCH

L.A. Marathon
(Los Angeles, California)
310-444-5544
lamarathon.com

Napa Valley Marathon
(Napa, California)
707-255-2609
napavalleymarathon.org

Shamrock Marathon
(Virginia Beach, Virginia)
757-496-5183
shamrockmarathon.com

APRIL

Boston Marathon
(Boston, Massachusetts)
617-236-1652
bostonmarathon.org

Country Music Marathon
(Nashville, Tennessee)
615-742-1660
cmmarathon.com

Spirit of St. Louis
   Marathon
(St. Louis, Missouri)
314-727-0800
stlouismarathon.com

MAY

Flying Pig Marathon
(Cincinnati, Ohio)
513-721-7447
flyingpigmarathon.com

Lincoln Marathon
(Lincoln, Nebraska)
402-435-3504
lincolnrun.org

Rite Aid Cleveland
   Marathon
(Cleveland, Ohio)
800-467-3826
clevelandmarathon.com

JUNE

Deadwood Marathon
(Deadwood, South
   Dakota)
605-642-2382
deadwoodmickelsontrail
   marathon.com

Grandma's Marathon
(Duluth, Minnesota)
218-727-0947
grandmasmarathon.com

Rock'n'Roll Marathon
(San Diego, California)
858-450-6510
rnrmarathon.com

JULY

Foot Traffic Flat
  Marathon
(Portland, Oregon)
505-525-1243
foottrafficpdx.com

Nova Scotia Marathon
(Barrington, Canada)
902-637-2760
barringtonmunicipality.com

San Francisco Marathon
(San Francisco, California)
415-284-9653
runsfm.com

AUGUST

Paavo Nurmi Marathon
(Hurley, Wisconsin)
715-561-4334
hurleywi.com

Quebec City Marathon
(Quebec, Canada)
418-694-4442
marathonquebec.com

Run with the Horses
  Marathon
(Green River, Wyoming)
307-297-0062
grchamber.com

SEPTEMBER

Road Runner Akron
  Marathon
(Akron, Ohio)
877-375-2786
akronmarathon.org

Rochester Marathon
(Rochester, New York)
585-264-1480
rochestermarathon.com

Toronto Marathon
(Toronto, Canada)
416-944-2765 ext. 501
torontowaterfrontmarathon
  .com

OCTOBER

Columbus Marathon
(Columbus, Ohio)
614-421-7866
columbusmarathon.com

Des Moines Marathon
(Des Moines, Iowa)
515-288-2692
desmoinesmarathon.com

Kansas City Marathon
(Kansas City, Missouri)
816-331-4286
kcmarathon.org

LaSalle Bank Chicago
   Marathon
(Chicago, Illinois)
312-904-9800
chicagomarathon.com

Portland Marathon
(Portland, Oregon)
503-226-1111
portlandmarathon.org

Twin Cities Marathon
(Minneapolis, Minnesota)
763-287-3888
twincitiesmarathon.org

NOVEMBER

Atlanta Marathon
(Atlanta, Georgia)
404-231-9064
atlantatrackclub.org

ING New York Marathon
(New York, New York)
212-423-2249
ingnycmarathon.org

Philadelphia Marathon
(Philadelphia,
   Pennsylvania)
215-685-0054
philadelphiamarathon.com

San Antonio Marathon
(San Antonio, Texas)
210-246-9652
samarathon.org

DECEMBER

California International
   Marathon
(Sacramento, California)
916-983-4622
runcim.org

Dallas White Rock
(Dallas, Texas)
972-943-4696
runtherock.com

Rocket City Marathon
(Huntsville, Alabama)
256-650-7063
runrocketcity.com

(Ralph Thompson, who has run marathons in each of the 50 states and more than 180 total, helped compile this list.)

By picking a fast marathon course you increase your chances—even stack the deck in your favor—of completing a marathon in **4 hours**.

Good luck and good training!

INDEX